Keto Desserts Cookbook

The Complete Ketogenic Desserts Cookbook with Easy, Delicious, & Low-Carb Recipes for Weight Loss, Lower Cholesterol and Boost Energy

Table of Contents

Introduction

Congratulations on purchasing your copy of *Keto Desserts Cookbook: The Complete Ketogenic Desserts Cookbook with Easy, Delicious, & Low-Carb Recipes for Weight Loss, Lower Cholesterol and Boost Energy,* and thank you for doing so.

I'm glad that you have chosen to take this opportunity to welcome the Keto diet into your life. I'm sure this book will help you find all the information and tools you need to better integrate the Keto diet plan with your habits.

Also, I thought I would share with you some delicious ideas and recipes for all tastes and for the best of your low carb diet, which I hope you will appreciate.

I'm going to show you a series of tricks and tips will help you prepare a healthy variety of sweets.

You can enjoy yourself with delightful Cakes, Muffins, Cookies, Brownies, Bar Recipes, Ice Creams, Ice Pops, Frozen Desserts, Tarts, Pies, Shakes and Smoothies.

You will find hundreds of easy to realize ideas that will best suit your situation or your needs at the moment, with all the preparation time, amount of servings, and the list of all the nutritional values you'll need.

You will also find lots of useful tips that will help you save money and time, and all the tools you will need to start making your favorite desserts.

Chapter 1: Overview of The Ketogenic Diet

The Ketogenic Diet may be a high-fat, enough protein, low-carbohydrate diet primarily employed in medicine to treat difficult-to-control (refractory) epilepsy in children. Diet forces the body to burn fat instead of carbohydrates. Generally, the carbohydrates contained in food are converted into glucose, which is then transported around the body and is particularly important in enhancing brain function. However, if there is little carbohydrate in the diet, the liver converts fat into fatty acids and ketones in the body. The ketone body enters the brain and replaces glucose as an energy source. Elevated levels of ketone bodies within the blood, a state is known as ketosis, result in remission within the frequency of epileptic seizures. About half of children and children with epilepsy who have tried some form of this diet have seen at least half of the number of seizures. So, the effect persists even after discontinuing the diet. Some evidence indicates that adults with epilepsy may enjoy a less effective diet, like a less strict diet, a modified Atkins diet. Possible side effects may include constipation, high cholesterol, slowing growth, acidosis, and kidney stones.

Keto Diet Basics

The basic therapeutic regimen for pediatric epilepsy provides only enough protein for body growth and repair, and enough calories to take care of the correct weight for age and height. The classic therapeutic ketogenic diet was developed in the 1920s to treat pediatric epilepsy. It was widely used in the following decade, but its popularity diminished with the introduction of effective anticonvulsant drugs. This classic ketogenic diet consists of a 4: 1 ratio of fat to weight to combine protein and carbohydrates. It is often obtained by excluding foods with high carbohydrates such as starchy fruits and vegetables, bread, pasta, grains, and sugar while increasing the consumption of foods high in fats such as nuts, cream, and butter. Most diets are made up of fat molecules called long-chain triglycerides (LCT). However, medium-chain triglycerides (MCTs) - from low-carbon chain fatty acids compared to LCTs - are more cryogenic. A variant of the classic diet, called the MCT ketogenic diet, uses copra oil rich in MCT, to supply about half of the calories. During this type of diet requiring less overall fat, a greater proportion of carbohydrates and protein are often eaten, leading to more food choices.

Epilepsy is one of the most common neurological disorders after stroke, affecting approximately 50 million people worldwide. It is diagnosed during a person's recurrent disease, unnatural seizures. These occur when cortical neurons fire excessively, hypersynchronous, or both, resulting in a temporary disruption of normal brain function. This can, for example, affect muscles, senses, consciousness, or amalgam. A seizure is often focal (limited to a selected part of the brain) or generalized (widely spread throughout the brain and resulting in loss of consciousness). The causes of epilepsy maybe for the spread; Some forms are classified into epilepsy syndromes, most of which begin in childhood. Epilepsy is taken as refractory (not yielding to treatment) when two or three anticonvulsants have not controlled it. About 60% of patients receive control of their epilepsy from the primary medication they use. In comparison, about 30% do not achieve control with the medication. When medications fail, other options include epilepsy surgery, vaginal stimulation, and, therefore, a ketogenic diet.

Diet In 1921, Rollin Turner Woodrat reviewed research on diet and diabetes. They reported that three water-soluble compounds, that-hydroxybutyrate, acetoacetate, and acetone (collectively known as the ketone body), were produced by the liver as otherwise healthy people once starved or were reduced Used carbohydrate, high-fat diet. Dr. at Mayo Clinic Russell Morse Wilder built on this research and coined the term "ketogenic diet" to explain a diet that produced high levels of ketones within the blood (ketonemia) through fat and carbohydrate depletion. Wilder hoped to get the benefits of fasting during a dietary therapy that would be maintained indefinitely. His trial on a pair of epilepsy patients in 1921 was the primary use of the ketogenic diet as a treatment for epilepsy.

Wilder's colleague, pediatrician Myanna Gustav Peterman, later devised the classic diet, which included 1 gram of protein per kilogram in children, 10–15 grams of carbohydrate per day, and therefore the ratio of fat to calorie balance. The addition of Peterman in the 1920s established techniques for the induction and maintenance of the diet. Peterman documented positive effects (improved alertness, behavior, and sleep) and adverse effects (nausea and vomiting for greater nausea). Diet proved to be very successful in children: Peterman reported in 1925 that 95% of the 37 young patients had improved dietary control and 60% had relieved seizures. By 1930, the diet was studied in 100 adolescents and adults. Clifford Joseph Barbara, Sr. from the Mayo Clinic, also reported that 56% of these older patients had improved diet and 12% became seizure-free. Although adult results are almost like modern studies of youth, they did not compare to contemporary studies. Barbara concluded that adults were least likely to benefit from the diet. Therefore, the use of the ketogenic diet in adults was not studied again until 1999.

MCT Diet In the 1960s, medium-chain triglycerides (MCT) were found to supply more ketones. Energy per unit compared to normal dietary fat (which are mostly long-chain triglycerides). MCTs are absorbed more efficiently and are rapidly transported to the liver via the liver vascular system rather than the system lymphatic. The severe carbohydrate restriction of the classic ketogenic diet made it difficult for people to supply delicious food that their children would have to bear. In 1971, Peter Hutten ocher designed a ketogenic diet, where approximately 60% of calories came from MCT oil, and this allowed for more protein and 3 times the maximum carbohydrate due to the classic ketogenic diet. The oil is mixed with at least twice the amount of skim milk, cooled, and peeled during meals or added to food. He tested it on 12 children and adolescents with different seizures. Most youths experienced both seizure control and improved application, with results that were almost like those of the classic ketogenic diet. Gastrointestinal upset was a drag, which prompted a patient to skip the diet. Still, the food was easier to organize and was better accepted by the youth. The MCT diet replaced the classic ketogenic diet in many hospitals, although some prepared diets that were a mixture of 2.

The revived ketogenic diet gained national media exposure within the US in October 1994, when NBC's Dateline television program reported the case of Charlie Abraham, son of Hollywood producer Jim Abraham. The two-year-old suffered from epilepsy that had remained uncontrolled with mainstream and alternative treatments. Abraham discovered the ketogenic diet in the epilepsy guide for people, and Charlie at John Hopkins Hospital to John M. Brought to Freeman, who had continued medical supplies. Under the diet, Charlie's epilepsy was rapidly controlled, and his developmental progress resumed. This prompted Abrams to market diet and fund research to the Charlie Foundation. A multilevel prospective study began in 1994, and the results were presented to the American Epilepsy Society in 1996 and published in 1998. There was an explosion of scientific interest within the diet. In 1997, Abraham produced a TV film: "First Do No Harm", starring Streep, during which a ketogenic diet successfully treats a young boy's arachnoid epilepsy.

As of 2007, the ketogenic diet was available from about 75 centers in 45 countries, and less restrictive versions, like the modified Atkins diet, were in use, especially in older children and adults. Ketogenic diets were also being investigated for a good treatment of epileptic disorders.

Efficacy

The ketogenic diet reduces seizure frequency by 50% in half of the patients who try it and up to 90% during one-third of patients. Three-quarters of the responding youth do so within a fortnight. However, experts recommend a minimum of three months of effort before it is considered ineffective. Children who have refractory epilepsy are more likely to benefit from the ketogenic diet than to try another anticonvulsant. Some evidence suggests that teens and adults may also enjoy the diet.

The Trial Designs

A preliminary study reported high success rates; In a study in 1925, 60% of patients became seizure-free, and 35% of patients had a seizure frequency reduction of 50%. These studies typically examined a group of patients recently treated by a physician (a retrospective study) and selected patients who had successfully maintained dietary restrictions. However, these studies are difficult to match with modern tests. One reason is that these older trials suffered from selection bias, as they excluded patients who were unable to initiate or maintain a diet and thus were selected from patients who would produce better results. To control this bias, modern study design prioritizes a prospective cohort (patients are selected before the start of the study), during which results are presented for all patients, regardless of the treatment they started. Or not (be known) as intent-to-behavior analysis).

Another difference between old and new studies is that patients treated with a ketogenic diet have changed over time. When first developed and used, the ketogenic diet was not a last resort treatment; Conversely, youth in modern studies have already tried and failed a variety of anti-collaborative drugs, so it can also be assumed that there is more difficult-to-treat epilepsy. Early and modern studies also differ because the treatment protocol has changed. In the old protocol, the diet was started at a fast pace, designed to lose 5–10% weight, and heavily restricted calorie intake. Concerns over child health and development led to the relaxation of dietary restrictions. Fluid restriction was once a dietary feature, but it increased the risk of constipation and kidney stones and is no longer beneficial.

Results

A study with a possible design for an intended treatment was published in 1998 by a team at Johns Hopkins Hospital and subsequently, according to a report published in 2001. As most studies of the ketogenic diet, no control group (patients did not receive the treatment) was used. The study enrolled 150 children. After three months, 83% of them were still on a diet, 26% had experienced an honest reduction in seizures, 31% had a spectacular reduction, and three were seizure-free. At 12 months, 55% were still on a diet, 23% had an honest response, 20% had a resounding response, and seven were seizure-free. Those who discontinued the diet from this stage did so because it was ineffective, very restrictive, or thanks to disease, and most of all, who were taking advantage of it. The two, three- and 4-year stakes still on a diet were 39%, 20%, and 12%. During this era, the most common reason for discontinuing the diet was because the youth became seizure-free or significantly better. In four years, 16% of the first 150 children had an honest decrease in seizure frequency, a staggering decrease of 14%, and 13% were seizure-free. However, these figures include many who were not on a diet.

Those remaining on the diet after this period were generally not seizure-free but had a spectacular response.

It is possible to combine the results of several small studies to supply evidence that is stronger than that available from each study - a statistical process known as meta-analysis. One of four such analyzes, conducted in 2006, conducted 19 studies on 1,084 patients. It is concluded that a third achieved a spectacular decrease in seizure frequency and half of the patients achieved an honest decrease.

The Cochrane systematic review in 2018 detected and analyzed eleven randomized controlled trials of the ketogenic diet in people who have epilepsy, for whom the drugs did not control their seizures. One in six trials compared to a gaggle assigned to a ketogenic diet with a gaggle not assigned to at least one. Contrast tests compared the types of diets or methods of starting them to make them more tolerable. Within the largest trial of the ketogenic diet with non-dietary controls, approximately 38% of youth and children had half or fewer seizures with the diet compared to 6% of those not assigned to the diet. Two larger trials of the modified Atkins diet had similar results when compared to a non-dietary control, with more than 50% of youth having half or fewer seizures with the diet compared to about 10% within the control group.

A systematic review in 2018 examined 16 studies on the ketogenic diet in adults. It concluded that the treatment was becoming more popular for that group of patients, that the efficacy in adults was almost like that of children, with the side effects being relatively mild. However, many patients abandoned the diet for various reasons, and therefore the quality of evidence to study children was inferior. Health issues include high levels of LDL, high total cholesterol, and weight loss.

Adverse Effects

A Ketogenic diet is not considered a benign, holistic or all-natural treatment. Like any serious medical therapy, it is going to end in complications. However, these are generally less severe and less frequent than anticonvulsant medication or surgery. Common but easily treatable short-term side effects include constipation, low-grade acidosis, and hypoglycemia if an initial fast is performed. Increased levels of lipids within the blood affect up to 60% of young people, and cholesterol levels can increase by about 30%. This will be treated by changes in the fat content of the diet, such as from saturated fat to polyunsaturated fat, and if consistently, by reducing the ketogenic ratio. Supplements are essential for combating dietary deficiencies of many micronutrients.

Prolonged use of a ketogenic diet in children increases the risk of slow or stunted growth, bone fractures, and kidney stones. Diet reduces insulin-like protein 1 levels, which is important for childhood development. Like many inhibitory drugs, the ketogenic diet hurts bone health. Many factors can also be involved, like acidosis and suppress somatotropin. Kidney stones develop in one in 20 children on a ketogenic diet (compared to one in several thousand for the overall population). A class of anticonvulsants called carbonic anhydrase inhibitors (topiramate, nonivamide) increases the risk of kidney stones. Still, a mixture of those anticonvulsants and, therefore, ketogenic does not increase the risk over diet alone. Appendicitis is treatable and does not justify discontinuing the diet. Johns Hopkins Hospital now supplements oral potassium citrate to all or any of the ketogenic diet patients, causing one-seventh of the occurrence of kidney stones. However, this empirical use has not been tested during a prospective controlled trial. Urinary stone formation (nephrolithiasis) is related to diet for four reasons:

Excess calcium (hypercalciuria) within the urine is accompanied by acidosis, thanks to increased bone disintegration. The bones are mainly made up of phosphate. The phosphate reacts with the acid, and therefore calcium is excreted by the kidneys.

Hypocitraturia: There is an abnormally low concentration of citrate in the urine, which normally helps dissolve free calcium.

Urine has a low pH, which prevents the acid from dissolving, resulting in the crystals acting as a nidus for the formation of calcium.

Many institutions traditionally restricted patients' water intake to a diet of up to 80% of daily needs] This practice is no longer encouraged.

Among adolescents and adults, commonly reported side effects include weight loss, constipation, dyslipidemia, and dysmenorrhea in women.

Maintenance

After Initiation, the child regularly visits the hospital outpatient clinic where a dietician and neurologist see them, and various tests and examinations are performed. These are held every three months for the primary year and every six months after that. Infants under the age of one year are seen more often, with the initial visit only after two to four weeks. A period of minor adjustments is important to ensure that consistent ketosis is maintained, and the patient is adapted to the meal plan. This fine-tuning is usually done over the phone with a hospital dietitian and involves changing the calorie intake, changing the ketogenic ratio, or incorporating some MCT or coconut oil into a classic diet. The level of ketosis in the urine is examined daily to determine whether ketosis has been achieved and to verify that the patient is following the diet. However, the number of ketones does not occur with an anticonvulsant effect. This is often done using nitro side-containing ketone test strips, which change color from barite-pink to maroon in the presence of acetate (one of three ketone bodies).

A short-term increase in seizure frequency may occur during the disease or if ketone levels fluctuate. If the seizure frequency is high, or the child is losing weight, the diet can also be modified. Seizure-control losses can result from unexpected sources. Even "sugar-free" food may contain carbohydrates such as maltodextrin, sorbitol, starch, and fructose. The sorbitol content of suntan lotion and other skincare products may also be enough to be absorbed through the skin and thus negate ketosis.

Discontinued

About 20% of Ketogenic diet youth are free from seizures, and many are ready to reduce the use of anticonvulsant drugs or eliminate them. Typically, the diet can be gradually discontinued over two or three months, about two years on a diet, or six months after being seizure-free. This is often done by lowering the ketogenic ratio until urinary ketosis is detected, then lifting all calorie restrictions. This time and method of dissection mimic anticonvulsant therapy in children, where the child has become seizure-free. When a diet is required to treat certain metabolic diseases, the duration is going to belong. The duration of the entire diet ranges from the treatment of the ketogenic diet team and parents; Studies of up to 12 years are situated and beneficial.

Children who discontinue the diet after attaining freedom of seizure have some 20% risk of seizures. The length of your time until repetition is very variable, but two years on average. This risk of recurrence compares with 10% comparative surgery (where a part of the brain is removed) and 30–50% with anticonvulsant therapy. Of these, which is a recurrence, just over half of the seizures can occur either with anticonvulsants or on a ketogenic diet. Recurrence is more likely if, despite seizure independence, an electroencephalogram shows epileptiform spikes, reflecting epileptic activity within the brain, but is below the extent that a seizure would cause. Recurrence is likely to occur also if an MRI scan shows focal abnormalities (egg, in children with tubular sclerosis). Such children may remain on a diet for longer than the average, and young people with tuberculosis who achieve freedom of seizure may remain on the ketogenic diet indefinitely.

A Ketogenic diet is calculated by a dietitian for every child. Age, weight, activity level, culture and food preferences all affect the hotel plan. First, energy requirements are set at 80–90% of the recommended daily intake (RDA) for the child's age (high-fat diets require less energy than typical high-carbohydrate diets). Highly active children or people with muscle mobility require more food energy than this; Children require less water. The ketogenic ratio of the diet compares the weight of fat to the combined weight of carbohydrate and protein. It is usually 4: 1, but children who are younger than 18 months, older than 12 years, or who are obese can also be started in the ratio of 3: 1. Fats are energy-rich with 9 kcal / g (38 kJ / g) compared to 4 kcal / g

(17 kJ / g) for carbohydrates or protein, so fractions are smaller than normal on a ketogenic diet. The number of fats within the diet is often calculated from the general energy requirements and therefore the ketogenic ratio is chosen. Subsequently, protein levels are determined for the development and maintenance of the body. For every kilogram of weight, there is about 1 gram of protein. Lastly, the amount of carbohydrate is consistent with what allowance is remaining while maintaining the chosen ratio. Any carbohydrate in medicines or supplements should be deducted from this allowance. The entire daily intake of fat, protein, and carbohydrates is divided equally into food.

A computer virus, such as recalculate, may also be used to help generate recipes. Food often consists of four components: heavy light whipping cream, protein-rich food (usually meat), fruit or vegetable and fats like butter, oil, or mayonnaise. Only low-carbohydrate fruits and vegetables are allowed, except bananas, potatoes, peas, and corn. Suitable fruits are divided into two groups in which they support the number of carbohydrates, and vegetables are divided equally into two groups. Foods within each of those four groups can also be freely substituted to allow for variation without having to recalculate portion sizes. For example, cooked broccoli, Brussels sprouts, cauliflower, and green beans are all the same. Fresh, canned, or frozen foods are equivalent, but raw and cooked vegetables are different, and processed foods are another complication. Parents need to be precise when measuring the amount of food on an accurate electronic scale of 1 g. The child must eat a full meal and cannot have extra portions; any snacks should be included in the hotel plan. Small amounts of MCT oil may also be used to help with constipation or to expand ketosis.

Seizure Control

Although several hypotheses are suggested as to how ketogenic diets work, it remains a mystery. Disorganized hypotheses include systemic acidosis (high levels of acid within the blood), electrolyte changes and hypoglycemia (low blood sugar). Although many biochemical changes are known to occur within a patient's brain on a ketogenic diet, it is not known which of them has an anticonvulsant effect. The lack of understanding during this area is consistent with many anticonvulsant drugs.

On a Ketogenic diet, carbohydrates are restricted so they cannot provide for all metabolic needs of the body. Instead, fatty acids are used because of the major source of fuel. These are used through fatty-acid oxidation within the mitochondria (energy-producing parts of the cell) of the cell. Humans can convert certain amino acids into glucose by a process called gluconeogenesis. Still, they cannot do so using fatty acids. Since amino acids are required to make proteins, which are necessary for the growth and repair of body tissues, they cannot be used to supply only glucose. This can cause a stretch to the brain, as it is normally completely fueled by glucose, and most fatty acids do not cross the blood-brain barrier.

However, the liver can use long-chain fatty acids to synthesize three-ketone body hid-hydroxybutyrate, acetoacetate, and acetone. These ketones enter the body and are partially substituted for blood sugar as a source of energy.

Ketone bodies are possibly anticonvulsant; In animal models, acetoacetate and acetone protect against seizures. Ketogenic diet leads to adaptive changes to brain energy metabolism that increase energy reserves; Ketones are more efficient fuels than body glucose, and therefore the number of mitochondria increases. This may help neurons within the face of increased energy demand during a seizure remain stable and should provide a neuroprotective effect.

The ketogenic diet has been studied in a minimum of 14 rodent animal model seizures. It is protective in many of those models and features a different safety profile than any known anticonvulsant. In contrast, fenofibrate, not used clinically as an antiepileptic, exhibits experimental anticonvulsant properties in adult mice, like the ketogenic diet. This, along with those studies showing its efficacy in patients who have not achieved seizure control on half a dozen drugs, suggests a singular mechanism.

Anticonvulsants suppress epileptic seizures, but they neither curse nor prevent seizures. The occurrence of epilepsy (palatogenesis) may be a process that is poorly understood. A pair of anticonvulsants (valproate, levetiracetam, and benzodiazepine) have shown anti epileptogenic properties in animal models of palatogenesis. However, no anticonvulsant has achieved this during clinical trials in humans. Ketogenic diets have been found to possess anti epileptogenic properties in mice.

Dessert can be a course that ends the meal. Of course, there are usually sweet foods, such as confection and possibly drinks such as alcohol or liqueur; However, within the US, it is going to include coffee, cheeses, nuts, or other savory items, which are considered separate courses elsewhere. In some parts of the planet, such as Central and Western Africa and most of China, there is no tradition of a dessert course for the conclusion of a meal.

The term dessert can apply to many pastries, such as biscuits, cakes, cookies, custard, gelatin, ice creams, pastries, pies, puddings, sweet soups, and tarts. The fruit is also commonly found in dessert courses because of its sweetness. Some cultures sweeten foods that are more common for making sweets.

The Ketogenic diet can be a very low-carb, high-fat diet that shares many similarities with the Atkins and low-carb diets. This includes reducing carbohydrate intake and replacing it with fat.

This reduction in carbs puts your body in a metabolic state called ketosis. When this happens, your body becomes incredibly efficient at burning fat for energy.

It converts fat into ketones within the liver, which can supply energy for the brain. Ketogenic diets can drastically decrease blood sugar and insulin levels. This, along with increased ketones, has many health benefits.

Different Types of Ketogenic Diet

There are Ketogenic diets in several versions, including:

- Standard Ketogenic diet (SKD): These are often low carb, medium protein, and high-fat diets. It usually contains 75% fat, 20% protein, and only 5% carb.
- Cyclic Ketogenic Diet (CKD): This diet consists of high-carb diets like 5-ketogenic days followed by 2-carb-days.
- Targeted Ketogenic Diet (TKD): This diet allows you to carbs around workouts.
- High-protein Ketogenic diet: This is often a typical ketogenic diet but involves more protein. The ratio is usually 60% fat, 35% protein, and 5% carb.

However, only quality and high-protein Ketogenic diets are extensively studied. Cyclic or targeted Ketogenic diets are more advanced methods and are mainly employed by bodybuilders or athletes.

A Ketogenic diet is less efficient for the disease and fewer risk factors. Research suggests that ketogenic diets are generally better than recommended diets. What's more, the diet is so full that you can simply track your food intake without counting calories. One study found that people on a ketogenic diet lost 2.2 times more weight than a calorie-restricted diet. There was also an improvement in triglyceride and HDL cholesterol levels. Another study found that people on the ketogenic diet lost 3 times more weight than the diet suggested by Diabetes UK. There are several reasons that a ketogenic diet is better than a diet, in which the number of protein increases, which provides many benefits. Increased ketones, low blood sugar levels, and improved insulin sensitivity may also play an important role.

Ketogenic Diet for Diabetes and Prediabetes
Diabetes is characterized by changes in metabolism, high blood sugar, and impaired insulin function. The Ketogenic diet can help you lose excess fat, which is closely associated with type 2 diabetes, prebiotics, and metabolic syndrome. One study found that the ketogenic diet improved insulin sensitivity by 75%. Another study in people with type 2 diabetes found that 7 out of 21 participants were ready to stop using all diabetes drugs. In yet another study, the ketogenic group lost 24.4 pounds (11.1 kg),

compared to fifteen .2 pounds (6.9 kg) within the high carb group. This is often a significant advantage when considering the link between weight and sort 2 diabetes. Additionally, 95.2% of the ketogenic group were ready to stop or reduce diabetes medication, compared to 62% within the high-carb group.

Keto's Health Benefits

Ketogenic diets originated as a tool to treat neurological diseases such as epilepsy.

Studies have now shown that the diet can have benefits for a wide variety of health conditions:

Heart Disease: Ketogenic diets can improve body fat, HDL cholesterol levels, vital signs and risk factors such as blood sugar.

Cancer: Keto diet is currently being used for many types of cancer and slow tumor growth.

Alzheimer's Disease: Keto diet can reduce the symptoms of Alzheimer's disease and slow its progression.

Epilepsy: Research has shown that a ketogenic diet can drastically reduce seizures in epileptic children.

Parkinson's Disease: A study found that the diet helped improve symptoms of paralysis agitation.

Polycystic Ovary Syndrome: Ketogenic diet can help reduce insulin levels, which may play an important role in polycystic ovary syndrome.

Brain Injuries: An animal study found that diet can reduce aid and aid recovery that occurs after brain injury.

Acne: Low insulin levels and eating less sugar or processed foods can help improve acne.

Chapter 2: Ingredients, Keto Dessert Essentials and All Tools you Need for Your Desserts

There are some main ingredients that are an absolute necessity in the Keto diet to get the right fat content you need instead of carbohydrates. You will find that these ingredients will be the new staple in your pantry, and your body will only be able to thank you.

Ingredients

Sweets usually contain sugar cane sugar, palm sugar, honey, or some type of syrup such as jaggery, syrup, chat, or syrup. Other common ingredients in Western-style desserts are flour or other starch, cooking fats such as butter or lard, acidic ingredients such as dairy, eggs, salt, juice, and spices, and other flavor-enhancing agents such as chocolate, spread, fruits, and nuts. The proportions of those ingredients, along with the methods of preparation, play a serious role within the consistency, texture, and flavor of the top product.

Sugar contributes to moisture and softness in food. Flour or starch components are proteins and provide a sweet structure. Fats contribute moisture and can enable the occurrence of crusted layers in pastries and pie crusts. Dairy products in food keep the sweets moist. Many sweets also have eggs, to help make custard or to grow and thicken a cake-like substance. Egg yolk particularly contributes to the richness of desserts. Egg albumen can act as a leavening agent or provide structure. Further innovation within the healthy eating movement has provided more information about vegetarian and gluten-free alternatives to quality ingredients, as a replacement for sugar.

Desserts can contain many spices and extracts to spread the flavor. Salt and acid are added to the sweets to balance the sweet flavors and to contrast the flavors. Some desserts are coffee-flavored, for example, an ice coffee soufflé or coffee biscuits. Alcohol can also be used as an ingredient to make alcohol desserts.

Ketosis may be a metabolic state characterized by elevated levels of ketone bodies within the blood or urine. Physiologic ketosis may be a normal response to low glucose availability, such as a low carbohydrate diet or fasting, which gives another energy source for the brain within the type of ketones. In physiologic ketosis, ketones within the blood are elevated above baseline levels, but the body's acid-base homeostasis is maintained. This contrasts with ketoacidosis, the uncontrolled production of ketones that occur in pathologic states and causes acidosis, which can be a medical emergency. Ketoacidosis is most commonly the result of complete insulin deficiency in type 1 diabetes or late-stage type 2 diabetes. Ketone levels are often measured in blood, urine, or breath. They typically range between 0.5 and 3.0 millimeters (mm) in physiologic ketosis, while ketoacidosis can result in blood concentrations greater than 10 mm.

Trace levels of ketones are always present within the blood and are increased when blood sugar stores are low. Therefore, the liver metabolizes fat acids mainly from carbohydrates. This increased carboxylic acid oxidation occurs during states of fasting, starvation, carbohydrate restriction or prolonged exercise. When the liver rapidly metabolizes fatty acids into acetyl-CoA, some acetyl-CoA molecules can then be converted to the ketone body: acetoacetate, beta-hydroxybutyrate, and acetone. These ketone bodies can also serve as an energy source as signaling molecules. The liver itself cannot use these molecules for energy, so the ketone body is released into the blood used by peripheral tissues, including the brain.

When ketosis is induced by carbohydrate restriction, it is sometimes referred to as nutritional ketosis. A low carbohydrate, medium protein diet that will cause ketosis has been named a ketogenic diet. Nutritional ketosis alone does not lead to ketoacidosis, and its safety is supported in trials of up to 2 years, although research on long-lasting ketosis is lacking. Ketosis as a treatment for epilepsy is well established and is additionally effective in the treatment of type 2 diabetes. Benefits are still under investigation during several neurological diseases, metabolic syndrome, cancer, and other conditions.

Supplements for Ketogenic Diet

Although no supplements are required, some are often useful, for example:

MCT Oil: Added to drinks or yogurt, MCT oil provides energy and helps to increase ketone levels. Look at several options on Amazon.

Minerals: Added salt and other minerals are often important when they begin thanks to changes in water and mineral balance.

Caffeine: It can be a benefit for energy, fat loss, and performance.

Exogenous Ketones: This supplement can help increase the Ketone level of the body.

Creatine: It provides many benefits for health and performance. It will help if you are combining a Ketogenic diet with exercise.

Whey: Use half a scoop of whey protein in a shake or yogurt to increase your daily protein intake.

Foods to Avoid

Any food that is high in carbs should be limited.

Here can be a list of foods that need to be reduced or eliminated on a Ketogenic diet:

Fragrant Foods: soda, fruit crush, smoothies, cakes, ice cream, candy, etc.

Cereals or Starch: wheat-based products, rice, pasta, cereals, etc.

Fruits: All fruits, except small portions of berries such as strawberries.

Beans or Legumes: peas, kidney beans, lentils, chickpeas, etc.

Rooted Vegetables and Tubers: Potatoes, sweet potatoes, carrots, parsnips, etc.

Low-Fat or Dietary Products: They are highly processed and sometimes high in carbs.

Certain Spices or Sauces: These often contain sugar and unhealthy fat.

Unhealthy Fats: Limit your intake of processed vegetable oils, mayonnaise, etc.

Alcohol: Thanks to their carb content, many alcoholic beverages can get you out of ketosis.

Sugar-Free Diet Foods: These are often high in sugar alcohols, which in some cases can affect ketone levels. These foods are highly processed.

Main Foods to Integrate

You should base the bulk of your food around these foods:

Meat: Meat, steak, ham, sausage, bacon, chicken, and turkey.

Fatty Fish: such as salmon, trout, tuna, and mackerel.

Eggs: Look for pasta or omega-3 whole eggs.

Butter and Cream: Look for weed when possible.

Cheese: Unprocessed cheese (cheddar, goat, cream, blue or mozzarella).

Nuts and Seeds: Almonds, walnuts, flax seeds, pumpkin seeds, chia seeds, etc.

Healthy Oils: Mainly extra virgin vegetable oil, copra oil, and avocado oil.

Avocados: Whole avocados or freshly made guacamole.

Low-Carb Vegetables: mostly green vegetables, tomatoes, onions, peppers, etc.

Spices: You will use salt, pepper, and various healthy herbs and spices.

Tools You Will Need

Most likely, many of these utensils, you will already have them in your kitchen; in fact, they will help you deal with your keto diet in the best possible way and will save you a lot of time.

The objects we are talking about are mainly:
- Electric Blender
- Mixing Utensils
- Whips
- Rolling Pin
- Fine Mesh Filters
- Mixing Base Plates
- Pans
- Baking Tray & Baking Dish
- Grills

In addition, if you already have a food processor, you will realize how useful it can be both in preparation and in cooking processes, making things much easier and saving you a lot of time.

Certainly, then you will need to combine the various baking paper or other non-stick systems to make cooking easier and especially in the subsequent cleaning of the various tools used.

Other easy to use tools are the predefined shapes or prints, to keep your biscuits, cakes and muffins in a uniform shape that will make baking more uniform and will allow you to have fun decorating your fantastic cakes in every way.

Benefits on Keto Desserts

One of my favorite parts about grocery shopping is that all the colors and shapes of the fruits overflow their wicker baskets within the produce section. That and, therefore, the perfect blend of sour and sweet that fills the air with aromatherapy that I cannot deny.

After the Keto lifestyle, it sometimes snatches the magic that fills my car with fruits. Including fruit within the keto diet can be a big controversy and one that you must deal with from every angle.

Fruits indeed provide great health benefits to the body, but an overdose can get us out of ketosis and prevent fat burning. Luckily, I did some deep digging to look for keto-approved fruits and sweets to satisfy the typical dessert lover.

I am willing to help you understand why carbs are limited in the first place so that you can understand why there are fruits. We are getting keto dieters to respond like watermelon keto has the most pressure. Then I will take you to avoid fruits and, therefore, to include the lowest carb fruits sparingly. Finally, you'll get 8 of the most important draw-worthy, fruit desserts to urge your fix. Let's dig

Why are Cars Limited on the Keto Diet?

The basic principle behind limiting carbs is that we would like our bodies to use fat for fuel, not sugar. Our bodies can run on 2 different fuels - one is that the sugar we get from carbohydrates and therefore the other is the fact that we get from healthy fats.

When we address high-fat low-carb diets, our bodies switch to using fat for energy. Once we refer to those energy molecules as "ketones", we become fat-burning machines with crazy brain fuel. This supercharged diet feeds our healthy brain fats from real fats like fish, eggs, good oil, and butter.

When carbohydrates break down just below the sugar, insulin triggers a craving and reward centers within the brain. But once we limit carbs and increase fat, we prevent unnecessary hunger and yearning in their tracks.

So, if high sugar and high carb intake exclude us from ketosis, what does this mean for fruits? Keto does not include high-carb / high-sugar fruits because their nutrients do not matter; our body still views them as sugar leading to a huge increase in our blood sugar levels. And this is the amount we want to avoid with the ketogenic diet. Insulin release and impaired blood sugar results in insulin are commonly referred to as "fat storage" hormones.

Insulin tells your body to "store this body fat and hold on to it with a lovely life," which causes the fat-burning to return to a frightening halt. Keto does the other. When our bodies enter ketosis, we break down fat and use it for energy - which helps us reduce it rapidly and effectively.

The good news is that even when fruits are limited on a ketogenic diet, we will still include some fruits and sweetened sweets, which will not exclude us from ketosis. So, let's go to therapy. I> Which way do you get the fruit of them thumbs and which one to bring down the thumb, what proportion will you have the way often which of them "getting to tell, and.

With sugar like Stuffed high carb fruits, mango, banana, grapes, pears, and pineapples are not a select keto. These fruits are very sugary and contain a lot of carbs. Dieters since keto have their daily carbs.

Chapter 3: Cookies, Muffins and Brownies Recipes

Keto Brownies

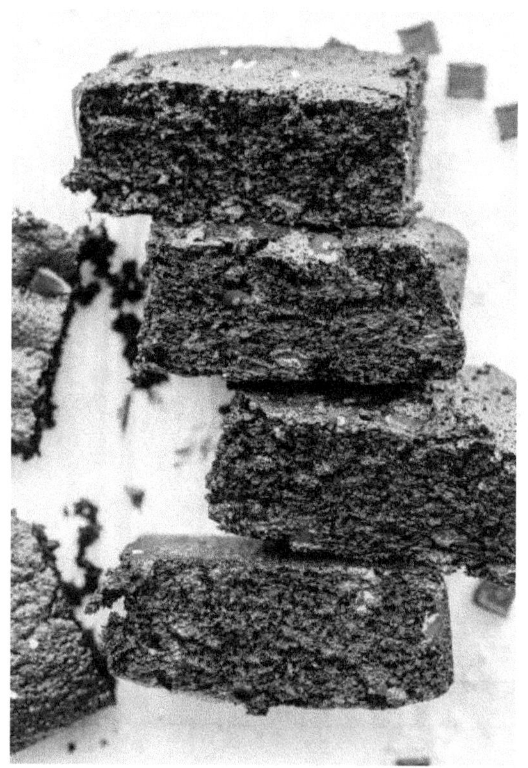

Ingredients

- 1 cup fine almond flour
- 1/4 cup chocolate
- 2 tablespoons Dutch cocoa or extra regular

- livers 1/2 tsp salt

- 1/3 cup melted copra oil or butter

- 3 tablespoons water or extra oil

- 2 eggs, or 2 Wax Eggs

- 2/3 cup Granulated Erythritol or Regular Sugar

- 1 tsp Pure Vanilla

Instructions

- Preheat the oven to 350 F. 8-inch pan or lined with parchment. Mix all ingredients well. Spread evenly in the pan. If necessary, smooth out, employing another sheet of parchment.

- Bake for 20 minutes on the middle rack, then let cool completely, and then they will still arrange.

- They organize even more if you are covered very little overnight. Brownies are delicious or without frosting). If you're trying a brownie, don't forget to leave a comment or rate the recipe below!

Keto Brownie Bombs

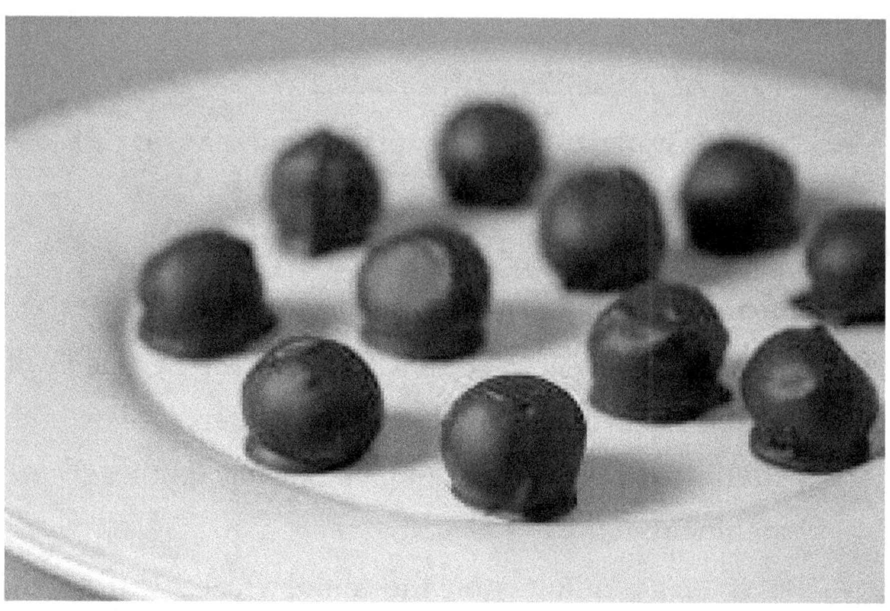

Ingredients

- 1 cup spread, or allergy-friendly
- 2/3 cup chocolate
- 4-5 teaspoon sweetener of choice, or desired
- 1/4 teaspoon salt
- optional mini chocolate chips
- optional 2 tbsp copra oil

Instructions

- Everything during a meal Blend the processor - scraping the edges as needed - until it forms a smooth dough.

- Roll into balls.

- If you have added melted chocolate or copra oil, just refrigerate until they are large enough to scoop into balls with a mini cookie scoop. I have not tried the recipe during a blender and am unsure if it might work, but if you experiment, then be sure to report back!

Keto Chocolate Chips Cookies

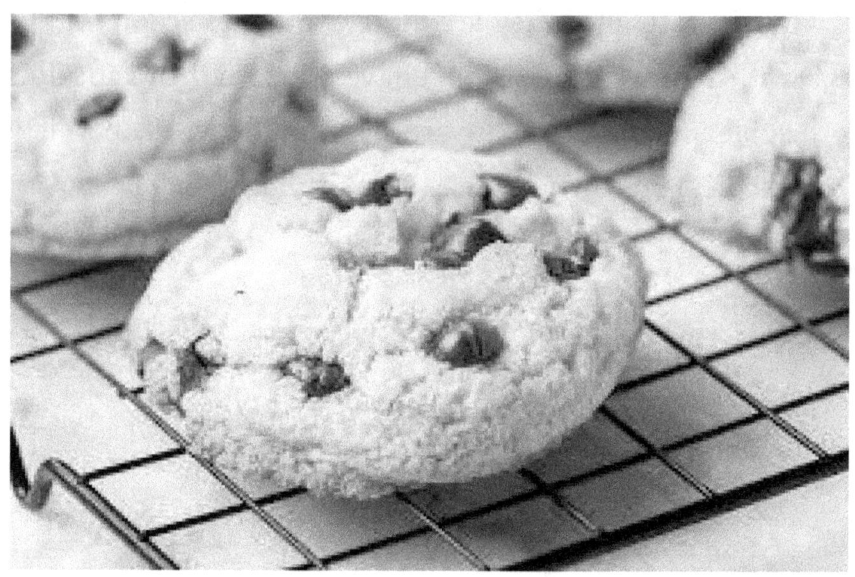

Ingredients

- 1 cup finely potato powder
- 2-4 Chopped spoon chocolate chips or sugar-free chocolate chips
- 2 tablespoons granulated sugar or powdered erythritol, or stevia equivalent
- scant 1/4 tsp salt
- 1/8 tsp soda
- 2 tsp copra oil.
- 1milksupply teaspoons pure
- 2-3 teaspoons Shoddy Vanilla, necessary

Instructions

- Preheat the325 F oven. Shake the dry ingredients thoroughly (so that you don't find yourself in a clump of baking soda!).
- Add wet to make the dough. Shape in Cookies - I first used a cookie scoop to make cookies, then shaped into cookies.
- Place on a cookie tray and bake 10-12 minutes on a middle rack.
- Allow cooling for 10 minutes before settling, as they are initially very fragile but arrange to cool once completely. If you are trying them out, leave a comment or rate the recipe below!

Coffee Cake Muffins

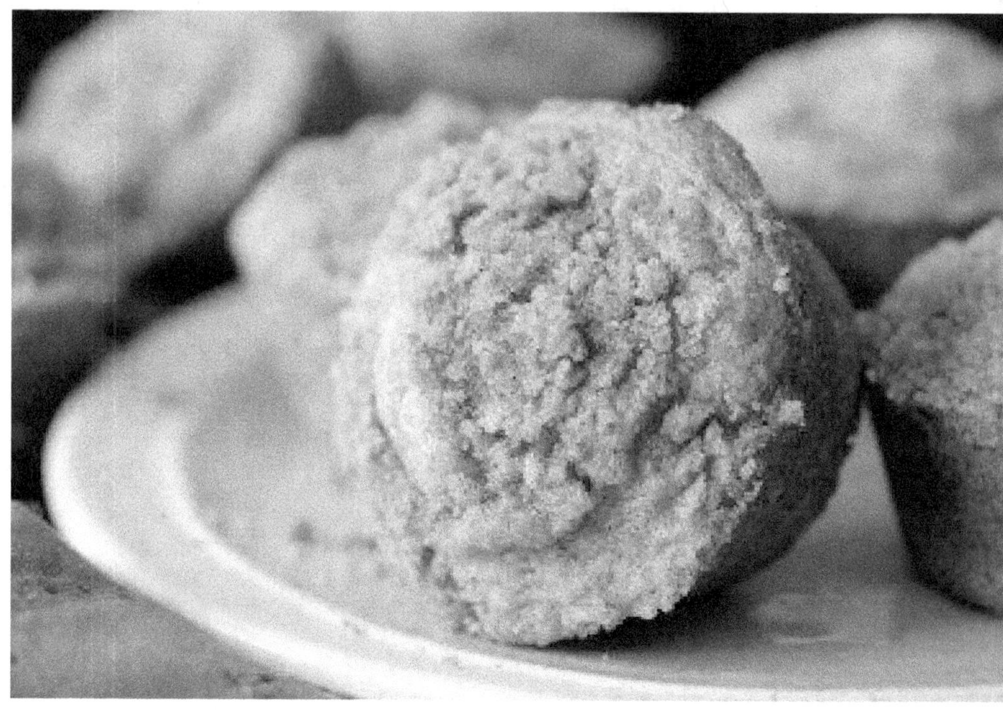

Ingredients

Batter:

- 2 tablespoons butter softened
- 2 ounces of cottage cheese soft
- 1/3 cup trim healthy momma gentle sweet or my sweetener
- 4 eggs
- 2 tablespoons vanilla
- 1/2 cup uncooked vanilla almond milk
- 1 cup almond

- 1/2 cup coconut Flour
- 1 TSP liver
- 1/4 tsp salt

Topping:

- 1 cup almond flour
- 2 tablespoons coconut flour
- 1/4 cup trim healthy mama Gentle Sweet or my sweetener
- 1/4 cup butter softened tsp melted
- 1 tsp cinnamon

Instructions

- Preheat three hundred- and fifty-degrees oven. Line a typical muffin tin with paper liners and spray with cooking spray.
- Combine all batter ingredients in a kitchen appliance. Mix well Divide among the prepared muffin tins.
- Combine the topping ingredients within the kitchen appliance and pulse until crumbly. Sprinkle over the batter.
- Bake 20-25 minutes until golden. If the crumb topping starts to insist, cover it with foil for the last 5 minutes.

Paleo Quick Bread Muffins
(Gluten-Free, Low-Carb)

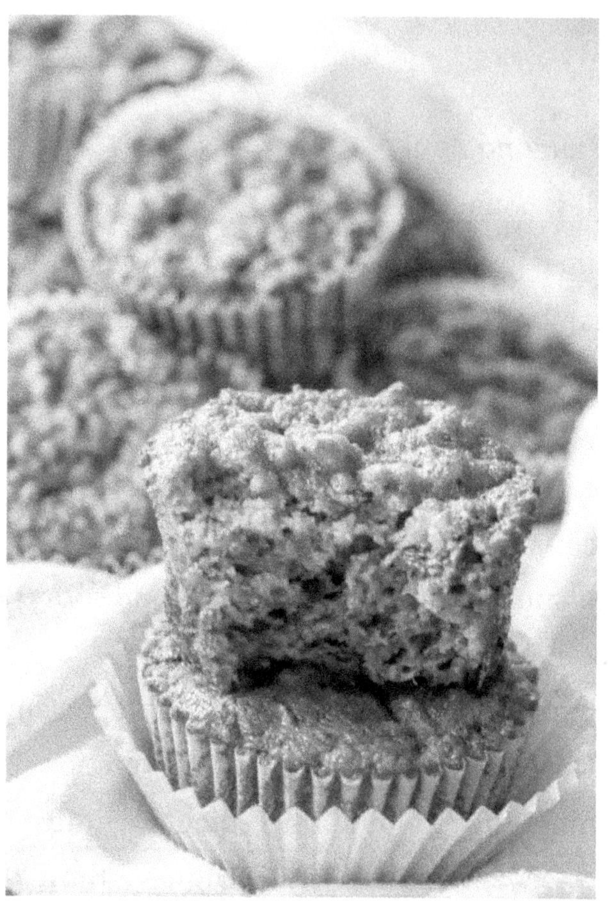

Ingredients

- 3 large eggs
- 2 cups mashed bananas 3-4 medium
- 1/2 cups almond butter spread can also be used
- 1/4 cup butter vegetable oil also used can be

- 1 teaspoon vanilla

- 1/2 cups flour, coconut flour, almonds can be used

- 1 tablespoon cinnamon

- 1 teaspoon Chios

- 1 of soda

- spoonful pinch of sea salt

- 1/2 cup chocolate chips optional and nutrition Sugandha Does not include

Instructions

- Preheat the oven to 350 degrees Fahrenheit. Line 12 muffin cups with liners; put aside.

- Combine eggs, bananas, almond butter, butter and vanilla during a large bowl. Until fully combined. Add coconut flour, cinnamon, chic, bicarbonate of soda and a pinch of salt. Stir with a wooden spoon until fully combined.

- Spoon batter into muffin tin, 3/4 full. Bake for 15 18 minutes or until golden. Chill for 10 minutes before removing from the muffin tin. Store in the refrigerator for 4 days.

Chocolate Spread Muffin

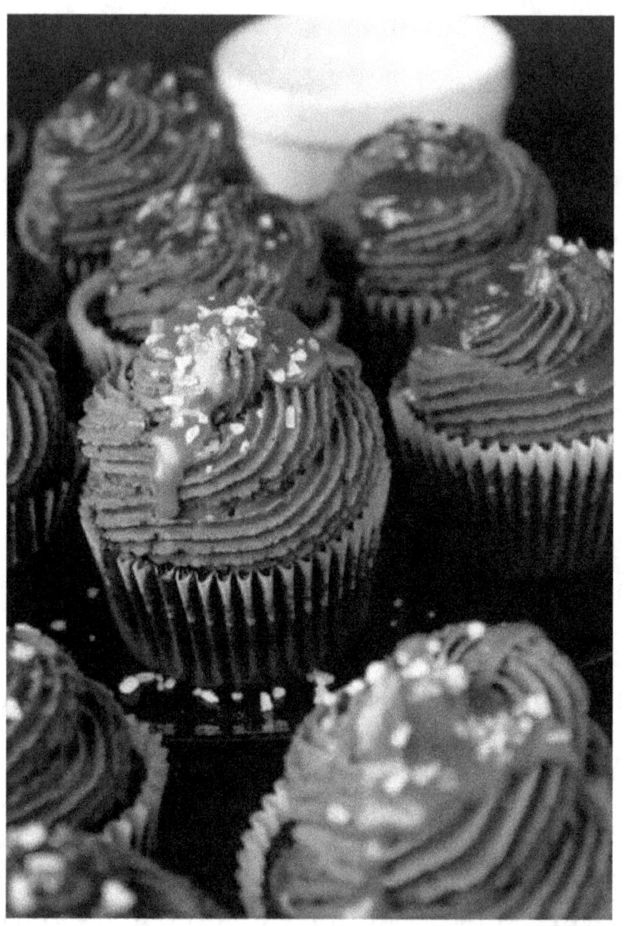

Ingredients

- 1 cup almond flour
- 1/2 cup nutritious erythritol sweetener spoon livers
- 1 pinch salt
- 1/3 cup spread
- 1/3 cup almond milk

- 2 large eggs
- 1/2 cup cocoa lime (or sugar-free chocolate chips)

Instructions

- Preheat the oven to 350 ° F and mix all dry ingredients (except the cacao) in a large bowl and shake.
- Add the spread and almond milk and stir to mix.
- Add in 1 egg at a time, until each is fully combined.
- Fold in cocoa nibs or sugar-free chocolate chips.
- Spray a muffin tin with vegetable oil spray and even distribute the batter to make 6 large muffins.
- Bake for 20-30 minutes and allow them to cool completely. Enjoy with some butter or a drizzle of sugar-free syrup.

Keto Pumpkin Spice Gourd Muffins

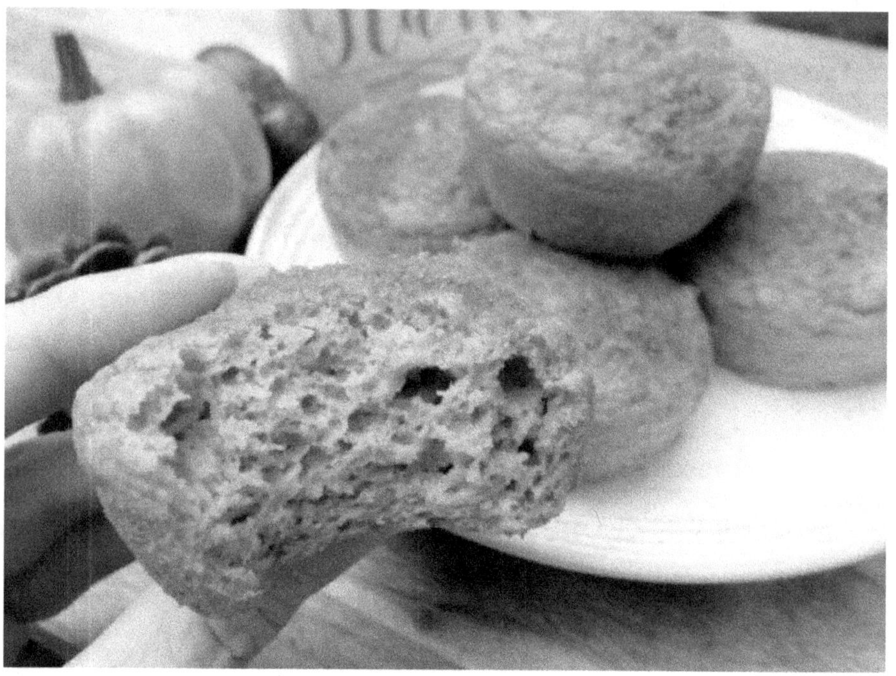

Ingredients

Dough:

- 2 cups chopped milk mozzarella cheese
- 2 tablespoons butter
- 3/4 cup superfine blanched almond flour
- 1/4 cup coconut flour
- 2 tablespoons yeast
- 3 tablespoons granulated erythritol sweetener teaspoon
- 1 cinnamon ground
- 1/8 teaspoon nutmeg

- 1/4 teaspoon Allspice
- 1/4 cup pumpkin puree
- 2 large eggs

Collector:

- 1/2 cup
- 2 tsp cinnamon
- salt over finch
- 2 tablespoons butter
- 2 tablespoons chopped pecans (optional

Instructions

Flour:

- Preheat the oven to 350. The degree is low.
- Combine the almond flour, coconut flour, yeast, sweetener, cinnamon, and nutmeg in a medium-sized bowl and mix well.
- In a large bowl mixes a couple of cheese and butter in. Stir well to microwave.
- Mixture for two minutes.
- Add the melted dry ingredients for the cheese with eggs and pumpkin puree.
- A rubber to make dough Stir well with Paula. Let dough sit for five minutes.
- Muffin tin with sleek Meanwhile butter.

To Assemble:

- Mix a small bowl sweetener, cinnamon, and salt and thoroughly blend Do it
- Pinch a small piece of dough and roll it into 3/4-inch diameter balls.
- Roll the ball inside the sweetener mixture and place it during the muffin cup containing ghee.
- Repeat with two more balls for a whole of three balls per muffin cup.
- Fill all ten cups with three coated dough balls.
- Add butter to the remaining sweetener and cinnamon mixture and microwave for 30 seconds.
- Stir and spoon a spoonful of the butter mixture over each muffin.
- Top with chopped pecans if in use.
- Bake within the center of the oven for 30-35 minutes, or until golden brown and slightly firm to the touch.
- Remove slightly and funky before serving hot.

Blackberry & Lemon Almond Flour Muffins

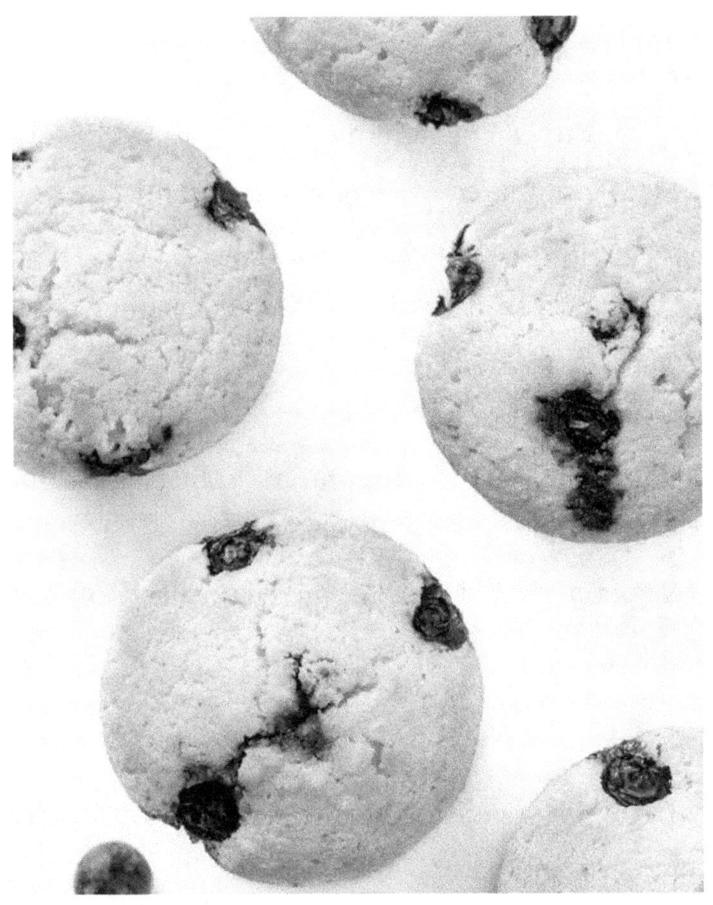

Ingredients

Blackberry Filling:

- 3 tablespoons granulated stevia/erythritol mixture (Pure) xanthan
- 1/4 teaspoonful
- 2 tbsp water

- 1 tbsp juice

- 1 cup blackberry for fresh or frozen

Muffin Batter:

- 1/2 cups Super Fine almond flour

- 3/4 cup granulated Stevia / Erythritol mix

- 1 teaspoon fresh lemon Khalkidhiki

- 1/2 teaspoon sea salt

- 1 teaspoon grain dryer

- 4 large eggs

- 1/4 cup Ancho Sector almond milk the original flavor

- 1/4 cup butter, melted, or copra oil

- 1 teaspoon vanilla is combined 1/2 teaspoon flavor. Mix the blueberry xanthan gum

Instructions

- 1 1/2-quart saucepan put together the granulated sweetener and so on. Add water and hence the juice one spoon at a time, whispering between additions.

- Stir in blackberry. Keep the pan on medium-low heat. Bring mixture to a boil, stirring often. Turn down the heat.

- Simmer, frequently stirring, until the berries are choppy, and a thick jimmy syrup is formed - about 10 minutes. Remove from heat and allow the mixture to cool.

For Muffin Batter:

- Heat the oven to 350ah Fahrenheit. Prepare a muffin pan lined with muffin paper.
- In a medium bowl, whisk together the almond flour, granulated sweetener, lemon peel, sea salt, and leaven.
- In a small bowl put together eggs, almond milk, vanilla, and flavoring. Stream in whispering butter.
- While stirring, slowly add the liquid material to the dry material.
- Spoon the batter partially into the prepared muffin cup, about 1/3 of the way. A depression within the batter within the cup using clean fingers or a spoon.

- Place one teaspoon of cold blackberry jam in each depression, dividing it evenly between cups.
- Cover the blackberry jam using the rest of the batter until each cup is about 2 / 3rds. To hide the jam, spread the batter on the sides of the cup that you like best. If there is a touch of 2 / 3rds filled in any case of cup batter, it is fine.
- Bake within a preheated oven for 25-30 minutes, or until spring when lightly touched.
- Cool any extras in an airtight container. They will also be frozen if they wish.

Low Carb Keto Chocolate Muffins

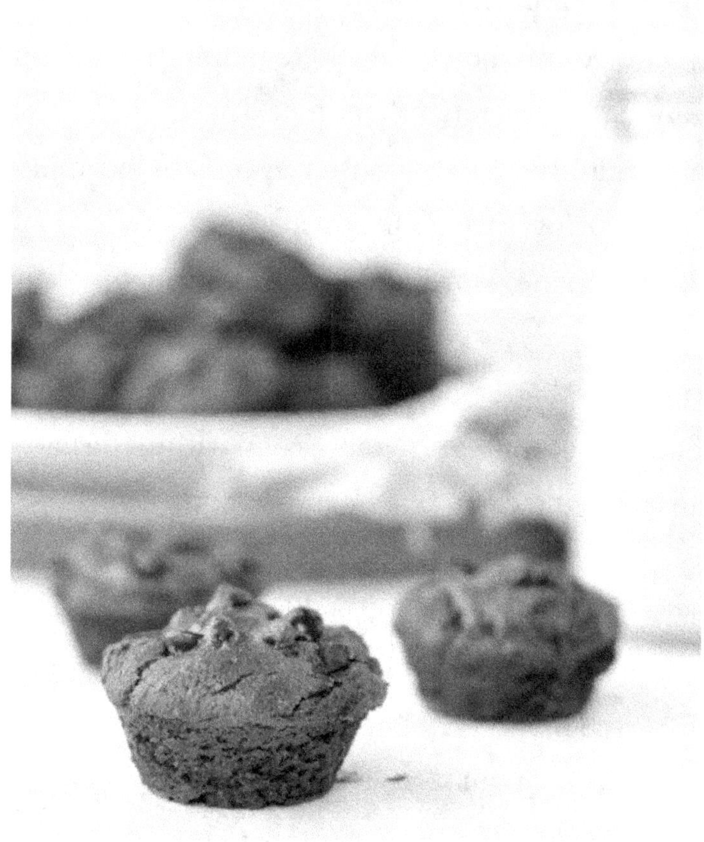

Ingredients

- 1/2 cup coconut flour
- 3/4 tsp soda
- 2 tsp chocolate
- 1/2 teaspoon salt

- 1 tsp cinnamon
- 1/2 tsp nutmeg tsp
- 3eggs
- 2/3 cup granular sweetener
- 2 tsp vanilla
- 1 tbsp oil
- 1 cup packed grated zucchini
- 1/4 cup cream
- 1/3 cup sugar-free chocolate chips

Instructions

- Line the oven preheats at 350F. Take 12 cups muffin tins with 9 cup liners and spray within the liners with a cooking spray of coconut flour, soda, chocolate, salt, cinnamon, sweetener, and nutmeg bicarbonate.
- In a separate bowl, mix eggs, vanilla, oil, cream, and zucchini.
- Add wet ingredients to dry and stir until combined. Fold inside the chocolate chips.
- Pour the solution into the muffin box with a spoon and bake for half an hour or until a toothpick comes out clean.
- Remove from the oven and allow it to cool within the pan.
- These keto chocolate muffins should be stored in the refrigerator for 1 week or see the note for freezing.

Blueberry Coconut Flour Muffins

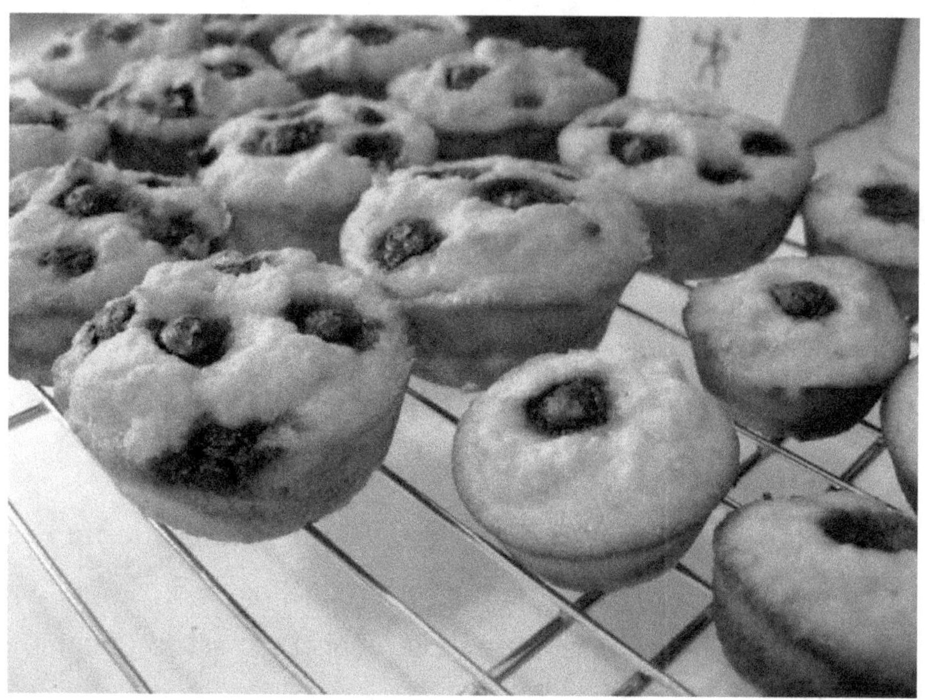

Ingredients

- 3/4 cup / 75 coconut flour
- 6 egg
- gram 1/2 cup / 100g copra oil melted
- 1/3 cup / 80ml coconut or almond milk
- 1/2 cup / 75 fresh mulberry
- gram 1/3 cup / 40 g granulated sweetener or more, to taste
- 1 teaspoon vanilla or flavored powder
- 1 teaspoon yeast

Instructions

- Preheat your oven to 180 Celsius / 356 Fahrenheit.
- Squeeze coconut flour into a bowl.
- Add all the ingredients aside from the blueberries and mix well.
- Stir within the blueberries, placing a few pairs to decorate.
- Line a muffin pan with paper cups and fill each cup in half with flour.
- Place the remaining blueberries on top of the muffins.
- Bake at 180 C for 25 minutes or until the top is golden brown.
- Notes For
- a nice light dough, you will separate the eggs and whisk the egg whites into hard peaks. After mixing the dough, fold it inside the egg white. Then add blueberries to the last.
- If you try to find out the "ego" taste in low-carb food, you will drop 2-3 egg yolk.
- You can use frozen blueberries; however, the fresh ones will hold together better and get less foggy.

Low Carb Cinnamon Bun Muffins
(Keto, Paleo, Vegan)

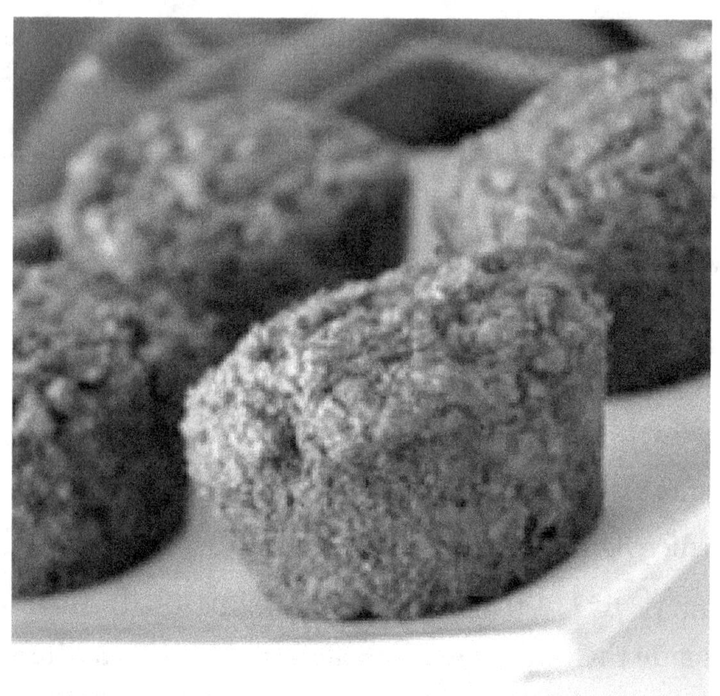

Ingredients

- 1/2 cup almond flour
- 2 scoop vanilla protein powder 32-34 grams per scoop
- 1 tbsp cinnamon
- 1/2 cup nuts or seed butter, spread, you can use edible seed butter, etc.
- 1/2 cup pumpkin puree, unripe apple, mashed banana or mashed sweet potato
- 1/2 cup copra oil

For Coconut Glaze:

- Butter 1/4 cup
- 1/4 cup milk Kadu
- 2 tbsp Juice

Instructions

- Heat the oven to 350 Fahrenheit and line the 12-count muffin tin with muffin liners and keep aside. It will also employ a mini muffin tin.
- In a large bowl, mix your dry ingredients and mix well. Add your wet ingredients and mix until fully incorporated.
- Evenly distribute the cinnamon bun muffin batter between the muffin liners. Bake for 10-15 minutes, put a skewer inside the center, check the 10-minute mark and see if it is clean. If this happens, the muffin is done. Allow chilling in the pan for five minutes, before transferring to a wire rack to cool completely.
- Once cooled, mix all the ingredients and mix the mixture until your cinnamon bun glaze is ready. Permit to drizzle and organize muffin tops.

3 Ways of Breakfast Egg Muffins

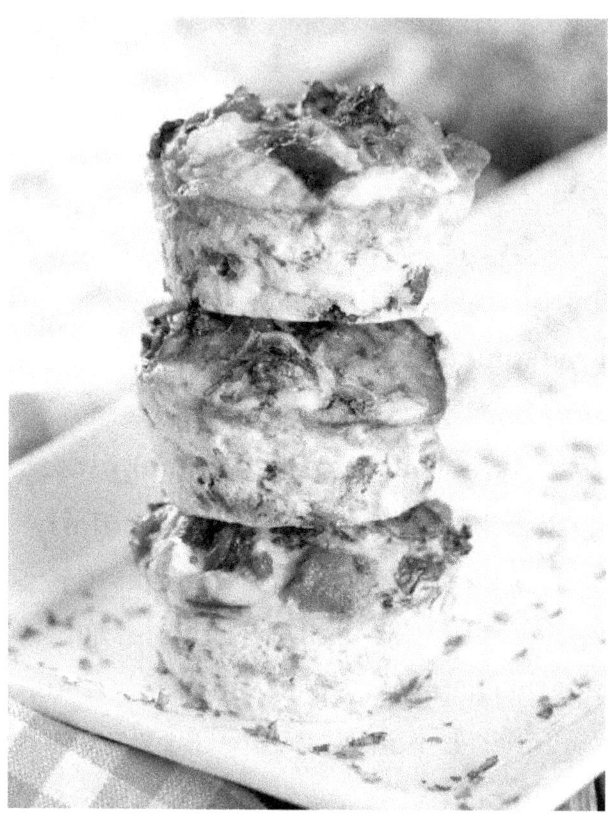

Ingredients

- 2 tablespoons finely chopped onion, (red, white or yellow/brown)
- salt and pepper, to taste

Tomato Spinach Mozzarella:

- 1/4 cup fresh spinach, roughly Chopped
- 8 grapes or cherry tomatoes, half

* 1/4 cup chopped mozzarella cheese

Bacon Cheddar:

* 1/4 cup cooked bacon, sliced
* 1/4 cup sliced cheddar

Garlic Mushroom Pepper:

* 1/4 chopped brown mushrooms
* 1 / 4 cup red bell pepper (capsicum), diced
* 1 large f Mc fresh chopped parsley
* 1/4 teaspoon garlic powder or 1/3 minced tablespoon garlic

Instructions

* Preheat oven to 350 ° F | 180 ° C. Lightly spray a 12-cup capacity muffin tin with non-stick oil spray.
* In a large bowl, combine eggs and onions. Season with salt and pepper to taste.
* Add half of the egg mixture to each tin of a mixed muffin tin.
* Divide the three topping combinations into 4 muffin cups.
* Bake for 20 minutes.
* Serve or store in an airtight container within the refrigerator for 4 days and warm when able to serve.
* Enjoy it!

Chapter 4: Ice Creams and Ice Pops Recipes

Butterscotch Coconut Cream

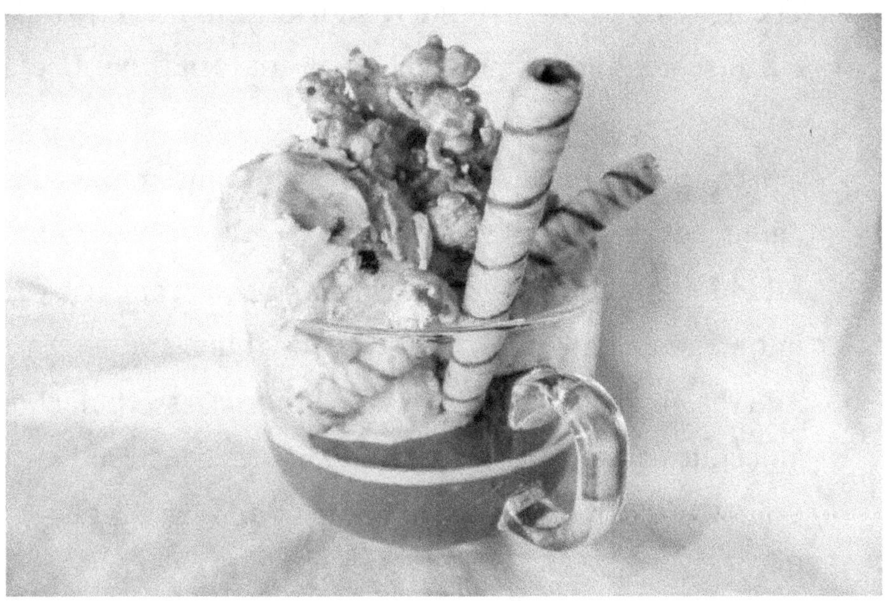

Ingredients

- 1 cup coconut milk (from a carton)
- ¼ cup sour cream
- ¼ cup heavy light whipping cream
- 3 tablespoons butter, browned
- 2 tablespoons vodka

- 2 tablespoons butterscotch flavoring
- 25 drops of liquid stevia
- 2 tablespoons erythritol
- ½ teaspoon xanthan gum
- 1 tsp sea salt

Instructions

- Coconut milk in a container, sour cream, cream, vodka, butterscotch flavor, sweetener, salt and Add the. Use an immersion blender to mix everything.
- During a pan on low heat, brown the butter to a dark amber color.
- Add butter to the base of your frozen dessert and use your immersion blender again to mix everything.
- Add the Frozen Desert Base to the Frozen Dessert Machine and churn according to the manufacturer's instructions.
- Enjoy! Add some chopped walnuts on top for a little extra flavor.

Brown Butter Pecan

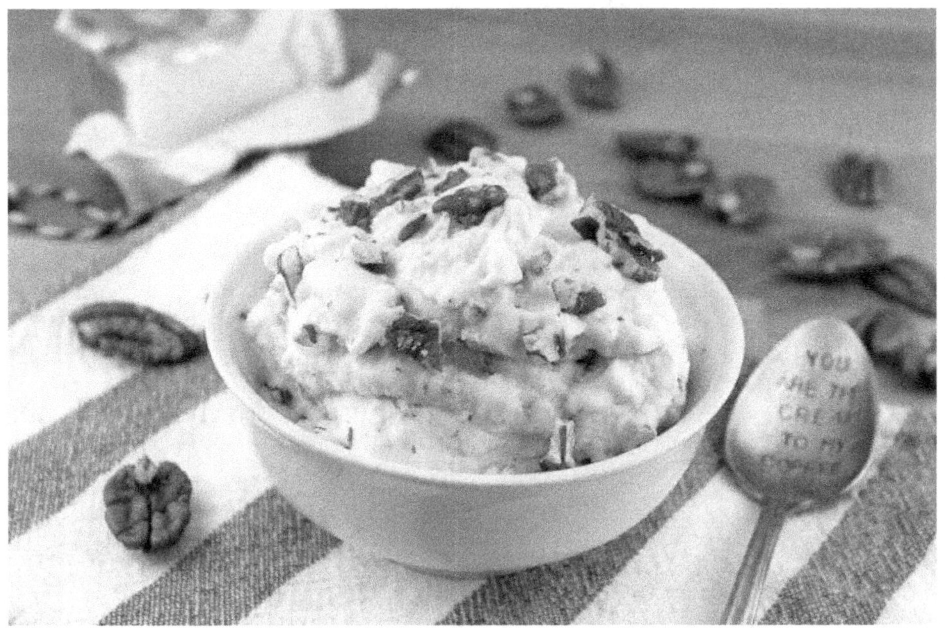

Ingredients

- 1 wet cup Unwanted Coconut Milk (from a carton)
- heavy cup heavy light whipping cream
- 5 tablespoons butter
- ed cups crushed pecans
- 25 liquid stevia
- ¼ tsp xanthan gum

Instructions

1. During low heat on a pan., Shake the butter until melted and begin to show a dark amber color.

2. Add pecans to a bag and crush the pecans.

3. Once the butter is browned, add cream, stevia, and pecans. Stir together

4. Put coconut milk, butter mixture, and xanthan gum in a container. Then use a whiskey to combine everything.

5. Add the mixture to your frozen dessert machine and run according to the manufacturers' instructions.

6. Serve and Enjoy!

Strawberry Swirl

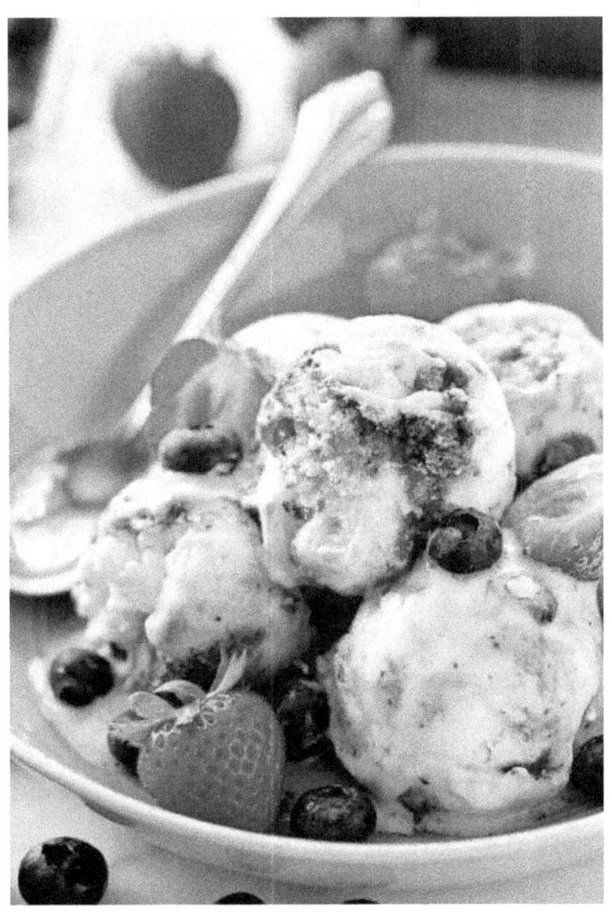

Ingredients

- 1 cup heavy light whipping cream
- 1/3 cup erythritol
- 3 large egg yolk
- half a teaspoon vanilla
- 1/8 teaspoon zinc gum

- 1 tbsp vodka

- 1 cup strawberry

Instructions

1. To heat, a cream set a pot with its cream on a coffee flame. Add 1/3 cup erythritol to dissolve.

2. Do not let the cream boil, just boil it slowly until all erythritol has dissolved.

3. Separate the 3-egg yolk from their whites in a deep bowl. Beat them with an electric mixer until they double in size.

4. Then, to temper the eggs so that they do not scramble, pour the eggs at once during a few tablespoons of your hot cream mixture.

5. Do this until the egg mixture becomes hot, then slowly pour in the remaining portion of the cream mixture, constantly beat. Add in some vanilla and mix.

6. This step is optional but helps the consistency of the frozen dessert stay creamy instead of ice - add one tablespoon of vodka and 1/8 teaspoon during xanthan gum.

7. Keep your bowl in the freezer for about 1-2 hours, stirring occasionally. If you have found a frozen dessert maker, be happy

to churn the frozen dessert according to the manufacturer's instructions.

8. When the frozen dessert is cooled and thickened to the touch, it is time to feature strawberries. Wash and shake a cup of strawberries and puree for 1-2 seconds without any. You will want the strawberries to be a touch chunky, with some juice to extract. We love our Antibullet for these kinds of tasks!

9. Add to the cooled cream within the strawberry mixture. Mix, but not mix over. You'll love the ribbons of strawberries you see in your vanilla ice cream!

10. Let this strawberry be immersed in frozen dessert chill for 4-6 hours or overnight. Then when you're able to enjoy, give a taste of frozen dessert on the counter for a minute or two and scoop! Enjoy it!

Keto Mocha

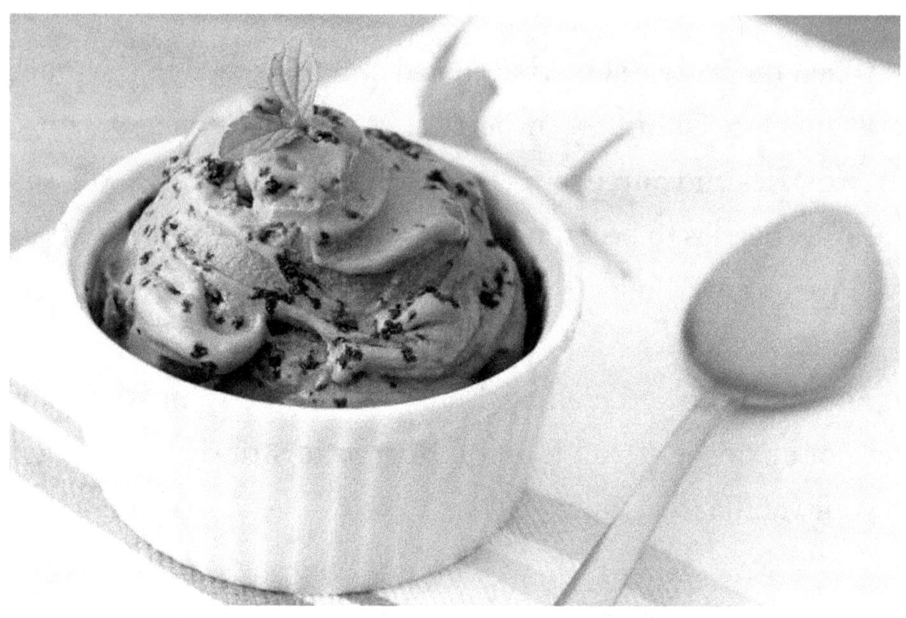

Ingredients

- 1 cup Coconut Milk (from a carton)
- cream cup light whipping cream
- 2 tablespoons erythritol
- 15 drops liquid stevia
- 2 tablespoons unsafe chocolate
- 1 tablespoon instant coffee
- ¼ teaspoon xanthan gum
- extractor cream

Instructions.

1. Glue in a container that will suit your immersion blender.

2. Use an immersion blender to make sure all ingredients are mixed well. Slowly add in the xanthan gum until a thicker mixture is formed. Add a much smaller amount than glue if needed.

3. Grow your frozen dessert machine, and follow the manufacturers' instructions.

4. Serve! You will add some extra instant coffee and mint to garnish.

Pumpkin Frozen Pie

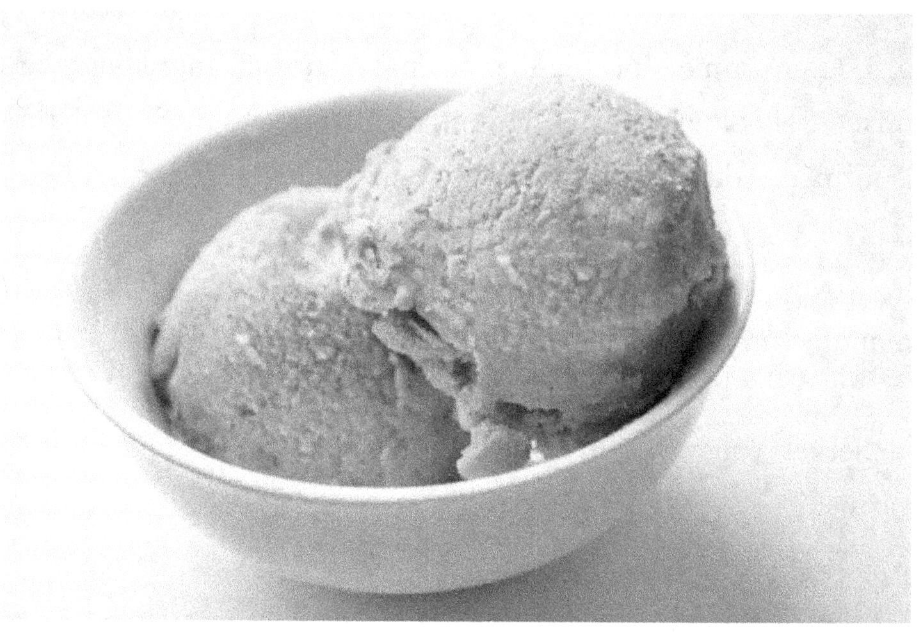

Ingredients

- Half Cup Pot Cheese
- Half Cup Pumpkin Puree
- 1 Tablespoon Pumpkin Spice
- 2 Cup Sweet Coconut Milk (From)
- Half Tablespoon Zinc Gumbs
- Cartoon 3 Egg Yolk
- 1/3 cup erythritol
- 20 drops Liquid Stevia
- 1 Tablespoon Maple Extract
- ½ cup chopped pecans, toasted

- 2 tablespoons salted butter

Instructions

1. Place on the stove with pecans and butter. Leave it on low heat so that the butter can turn brown. If you do not have pecans, place them in a pan, ground, and toast on low heat for about 7-10 minutes.

2. Place all remaining ingredients in a container that will house your immersion blender.

3. Using your immersion blender, mix all the ingredients into a smooth mixture.

4. According to your manufacturer's instructions, add the mixture to your frozen dessert machine.

5. Finally, once your butter turns brown and so the pecans have soaked several kinds of butter, place inside the frozen dessert machine.

6. Follow the churning instructions according to the instructions of your frozen dessert maker. Enjoy it!

Chocolate Chunk and Avocado

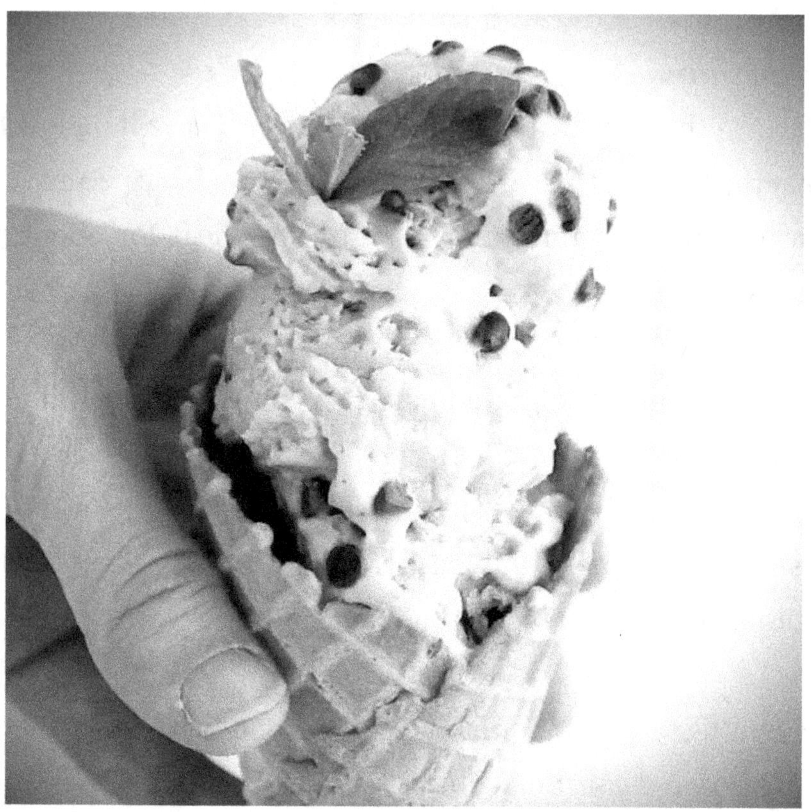

Ingredients

- 2 large Hass avocados,
- 1 cup coconut milk (from a carton)
- ½ cup heavy light whipping cream
- ½ cup sweet chocolate
- 2 tablespoons vanilla
- ½ cup erythritol powder
- 25 drops liquid stevia

- 6 squares baker's chocolate unsweetened

Instructions

1. Cut two avocados in half, then take out the avocado in a bowl.

2. 1 cup coconut milk (from a carton), 1/2 cup cream, and 2 tablespoons. Vanilla. Use an immersion blender to blend this mixture until smooth and creamy.

3. During a spice grinder, grind erythritol until it is powdered. Add erythritol, liquid stevia, and chocolate to the creamy avocado mixture and mix again.

4. Once the mixture is smooth, cut 6 squares of baked chocolate and pour it into the bowl. Use a spoon or fork to blend the chocolate.

5. Leave the bowl inside the fridge for 6–12 hours to cool completely.

6. About 15-20 minutes before you want to serve your frozen dessert machine and follow the instructions according to the manufacturer's notes.

7. You will store it within the freezer to harden for a few hours, but you will immediately feel soft serve. Enjoy it!

Keto Cookies and Crème

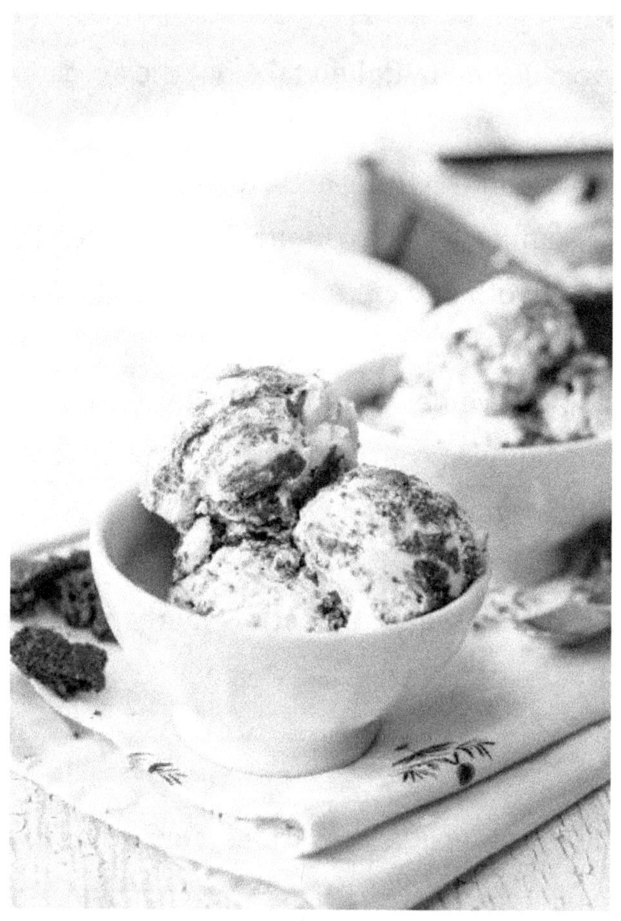

Ingredients

Cookie Crumbs:

- al cup almond flour
- ¼ cup chocolate ¼ cup
- soda
- a cup of cup erythritol

- ½ teaspoon vanilla

- 1 ½ tbsp copra oil, softened tsp

- 1, temperature

- salt Kamchatka

Ice Cream:

- 2. Cream

- 1 tablespoon vanilla

- cup Erythritol Mond

- cup almond milk spam

Instructions

1. Preheat 300F oven. Line 9-inch circular cake pan with parchment paper and spray with oil of choice.

2. Combine almond flour, chocolate, soda, erythritol bicarbonate and salt in a medium bowl until smooth.

3. Add vanilla and copra oil and mix until the mixture is ready into fine pieces.

4. Add the egg and mix until the cookie batter starts to stick together and form a ball.

5. Transfer the batter to the prepared cake pan and press the batter thinly with your fingers until it covers the rock bottom of the pan.

6. Place the pan in a preheated oven and bounce the center of the cookie back for 20 minutes or until it is pressed.
7. When the baking is finished, remove the pan from the oven and let it cool.
8. After the cookie cools, break the cookie into small pieces.

9. During a large bowl, whisk the light whipping cream with an electric mixer until stiff peaks form.

10. Add vanilla and erythritol, and whip until well combined.

11. Add the almonds to the milk and beat until the mixture thickens.

12. Transfer the cream mixture to the frozen dessert maker and until the frozen dessert begins to take its shape.

13. Slowly pour cookie crumbles while the frozen dessert maker is churning to mix crumbles evenly into the frozen dessert.

14. Once all the pieces of the cookie are included, transfer the frozen desserts into a gallon freezer-safe container and freeze for at least 2 hours before serving.

Low Carb Destiny Popsicles

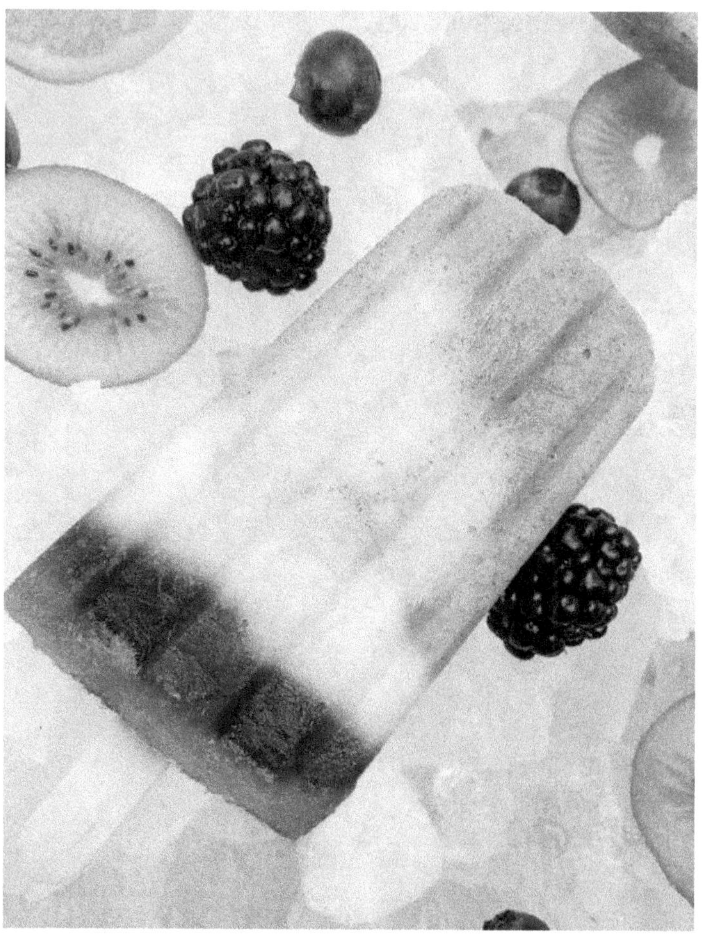

Ingredients

- 1 cup Dairy Pure Sour Cream
- 1 cup Heavy Light Whipping Cream Divided
- 1/2 cup Powdered Sweetener
- 1/2 Tsp Vanilla
- 1 cup Chopped Fresh Strawberries

- 2 Tablespoon Chocolate

Instructions

- In a large bowl, whisks together the sour cream. Whisk, 3/4 cup light whipping cream, sweetener, and vanilla until well combined.
- In a blender or kitchen appliance, puree the strawberries until smooth. Add 1/2 cup of the sour cream mixture and mix until well combined.
- Transfer 1/2 cup of the sour cream mixture to another bowl and pour within chocolate until smooth. It will be quite thick, so mix extra light whipping cream 1 tbsp at a time until it is thin and has a "spoon" consistency.
- Transfer the chocolate mixture to a frosting piping bag or an outer Ziplock bag and cut the very tip. Use the bag to pipe a fine layer into the popsicle mold, each about 1/3 full. As you try to create the layer, you will not get any drips while under the edges (as they are going to show the equivalent of your other layers).
- If necessary, use a Q-tip to wash the edges of the mold.
- Apply the leftover vanilla mixture over the chocolate, filling about 2/3 of the mark on each Popsicle mold (you can also pour it during a bag, or simply pour it from a measuring cup). Touch up the edges.
- Pour strawberries over the vanilla mixture, filling the highest (again, during a piping bag or by measurement) of

almost every mold. Add 2/3 of the wooden sticks to each popsicle and allow the firm to set for about 4 to five hours.

- To release, move the predicate on the molds and gently tug on the stick.

Sugar-Free Chocolate Popsicles

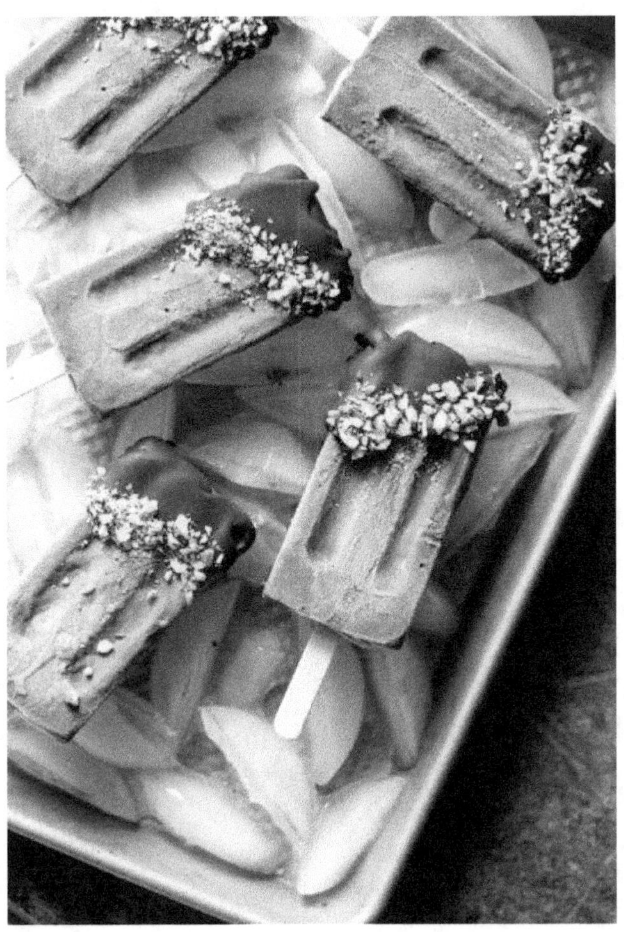

Ingredients

- Confectionery 1 cup heavy light whipping cream
- Extended1 tsp chocolate liquid stevia unsweetened
- 1.5 cups almond milk
- 1/2 cup fat no sugar
- 1/4 cup chocolate unsaturated in sugar

- 1 cup sugar-free magic shell optional

Instructions

- Hand Mix with or use a blender to blend all ingredients except for an optional chocolate coating. Blend for only a few seconds to mix the ingredients. If you mix for too long, the mixture will be like the cream within the recipe. Taste and adjust stevia as needed.
- Pour into popsicle molds and freeze for 2-3 hours or until hardened. Once hardened, hold the mold out under hot running water to facilitate release from the molds.
- Place popsicles on a parchment-lined baking sheet. Drizzle the chocolate coating or, if desired, spread the coating with a spoon on each side of the popsicle. Put back on the baking sheet to freeze again for about 10 minutes or overnight.

Keto Fruit Ice Pops

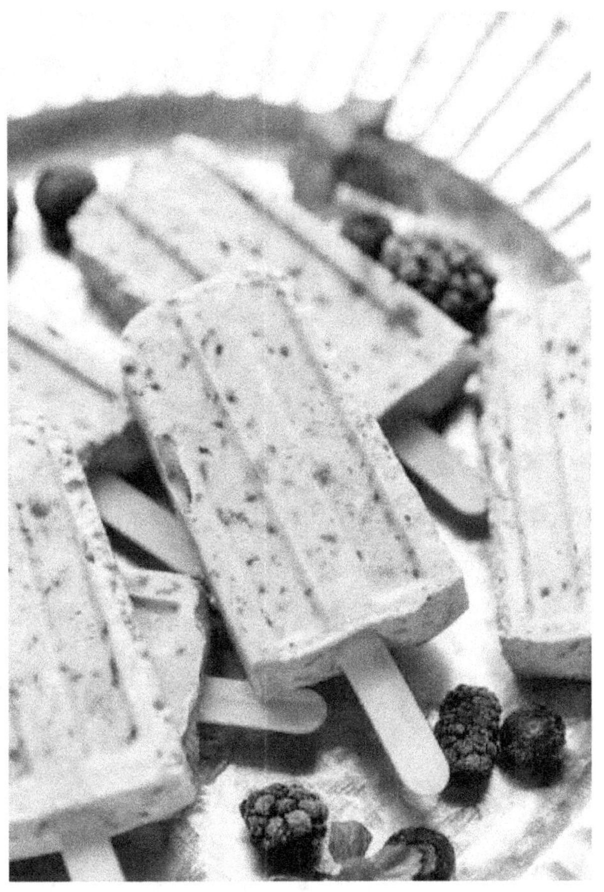

Ingredients

- 2 cups canned coconut milk
- 1/3 cup xylitol, erythritol or sweetener of choice
- 1/8 teaspoon salt
- 1 1/2 pure vanilla teaspoon or pasta flavor
- desired flavored ingredients

Instructions

- Coconut milk, not chat or coconut milk. If desired, you will use seeds from a flavor instead of extracts. To make keto ice cream: Stir the milk, sweetener, salt, and vanilla together.

- If you've got a frozen dessert machine, just churn it according to the manufacturer's instructions.

- Or to make it without a frozen dessert machine, freeze the mixture in a cube tray, then blend the frozen cubes like Vitamix during a high-speed blender or to mix them during a kitchen appliance or regular blender. Melt enough. Eat as is or freeze for an hour to a strong texture. Thanks to not having any preservatives or stabilizers, the Keto Frozen Desert is the best day it has been made. Still, you will technically freeze the leftovers for a month and melt before serving.

Chapter 5: Cakes and Bar Recipes

Chocolate Coconut Fuse Bars

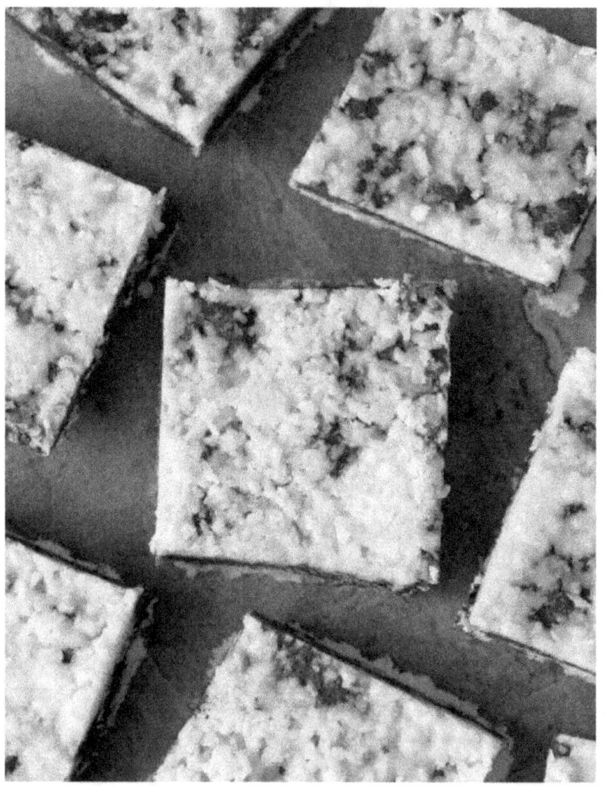

Ingredients

- 3 cups chopped uncut coconut (240 g)
- 1/4 cup sweetener (see note below)
- 1/2 cup melted copra oil or coconut butter (96 grams)

- 1/2 teaspoon pure vanilla
- 1 / 4 teaspoons salt
- 1 1/2 cups chocolate chips or sugar-free chocolate chips
- 1/3 cup almond butter, or extra chips or coconut oil/butter

Instructions

- You can either use 1/4 cup liquid sweetener (agave, honey, pure maple syrup), or you can use stevia. Add 1/4 cup of extra copra oil to make an equal sweetness and liquid spacing.
- Line an 8x8 pan with the parchment edges up. Combine the first 5 ingredients - I like to mix during kitchen tools, but this is often done by hand. (If discarding the kitchen appliance, you will raise the copra oil to 2/3 cup to make sure they are not uprooted. However, the strips within the photos would have been hand-mixed without additional oil. And still cut their size. So, it's up to you!) Spread the mixture into the pan about 2/3. Rather well depressed. Carefully melt the chocolate, dissolve in almond butter and pour over coconut when using. Sprinkle the remaining coconut on top and refrigerate for 1 hour or until firm. On quiet days or for indoor parties, bars are fine for getting away. Store leftovers in the fridge or freezer.

Keto Cheesecake

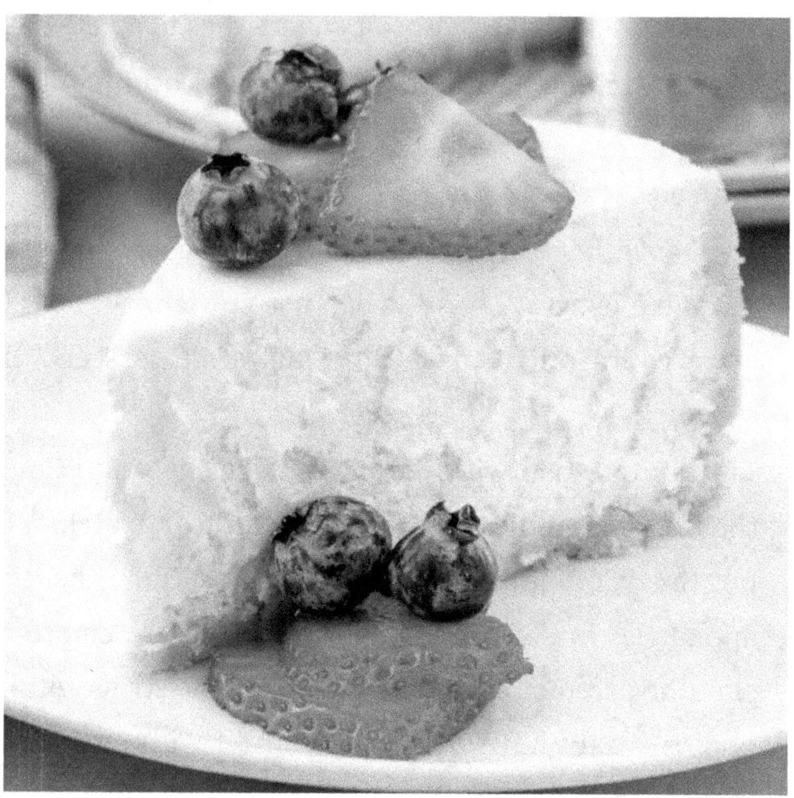

Ingredients

- 24 oz cheese or vegetarian cheese
- 2 cups yogurt, such as coconut milk yogurt
- 2 1/2 tablespoons pure vanilla
- 1 tbsp juice, optional
- 2/3 cup erythritol (sugar or syrup also work for non-keto)
- 1 / 4 cups almond flour

Instructions

- Feel free to use a shop-bought crust or make it crustless, or here is the crust I used: 2 cups almonds or pecans flour (you can use the dough to make), 1/4 tsp salt, 4-6 tbsp melted copra oil or enough water to make it slightly sticky). Combine all ingredients, pour into an 8 or 9-inch springform pan, press evenly, then set aside during filling.

- Preheat the oven to 350 F. Fill any baking pan about half full of water and place it on the bottom rack of the oven. Bring the cheese to temperature, then beat all ingredients during a blender or kitchen appliance until smooth (overeating can cause cracking as it bakes). I usually incorporate lemon for a classic cheesecake flavor. However, it will still work if you don't have one available and wish to get away.

- Spread on top of the prepared crust. Place on the center rack (top of the rack with the water pan). Bake for half an hour (or 38 minutes using an 8-inch pan), and do not open the oven at least during this point.

- Once the time has passed, do not open the oven, but turn off the heat and allow the cheesecake to sit in the oven within 5 minutes. Then remove from the oven - it will still look underdone.

- Let cool on the counter for 20 minutes, then refrigerate overnight, during which era it will be quite organized. As I mentioned within the post, cooling time is important, so the cake cools slowly and thus does not crack. Keep the remaining pieces stored in the refrigerator within 3-4 days or slice and freeze if desired. If you make it, make sure to remove the review or rate it below!

Classic Cinnamon Sugar Donuts

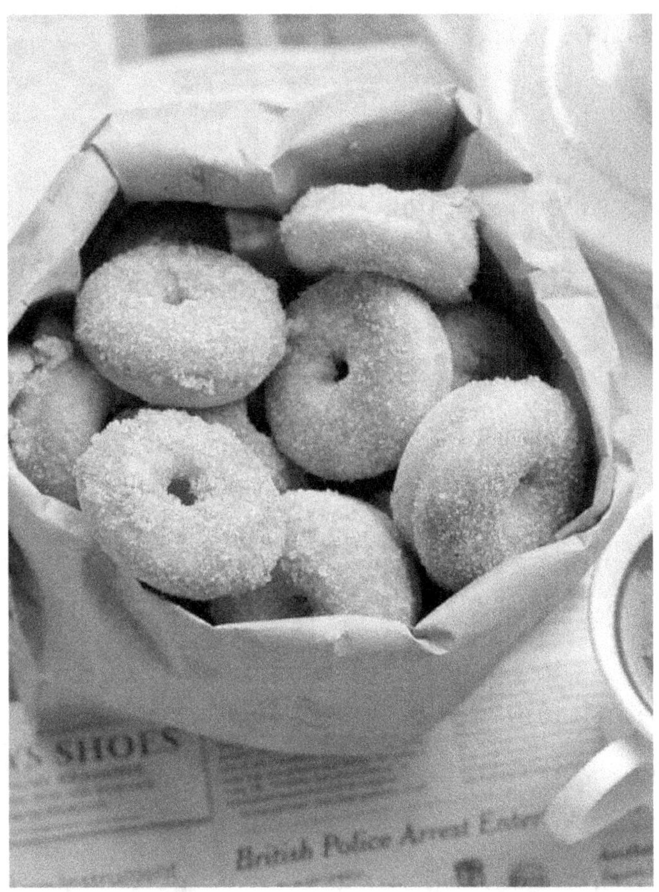

Ingredients

- Half cup creams
- 5 tablespoons butter, soft
- 2 large eggs
- 1 tablespoon vanilla
- half cup powder sweetener, Lecanto with code MELISSA20 20% discount

- 1 half-cup blanched almond flour
- 2 tablespoons psyllium husk powder
- 2 teaspoons lever
- 1/2 teaspoon nutmeg
- 1/2 teaspoon ginger
- 1/4 teaspoon sleeping
- for the covering:
- 2 teaspoons butter,
- 1 teaspoon cinnamon
- elated cup granulated sweetener

Instructions

- Preheat the oven to 350 degrees. Line a muffin pan with paper.
- In a medium bowl using an electric mixer, cream butter, sweetener, and vanilla until smooth. Hammer in eggs and cream.
- In a separate bowl, mix all the dry ingredients (except the topping ingredients) together. Slowly raise the wet material continuously with an electric mixer.
- The spoon also amounts to each muffin cup.
- Cook for 18-20 minutes or until the edges are golden.
- Let cool completely.
- Brush the finished muffins with butter, revealing the cinnamon sweetener mixture. service tax!

Cinnamon Walnut Katharine

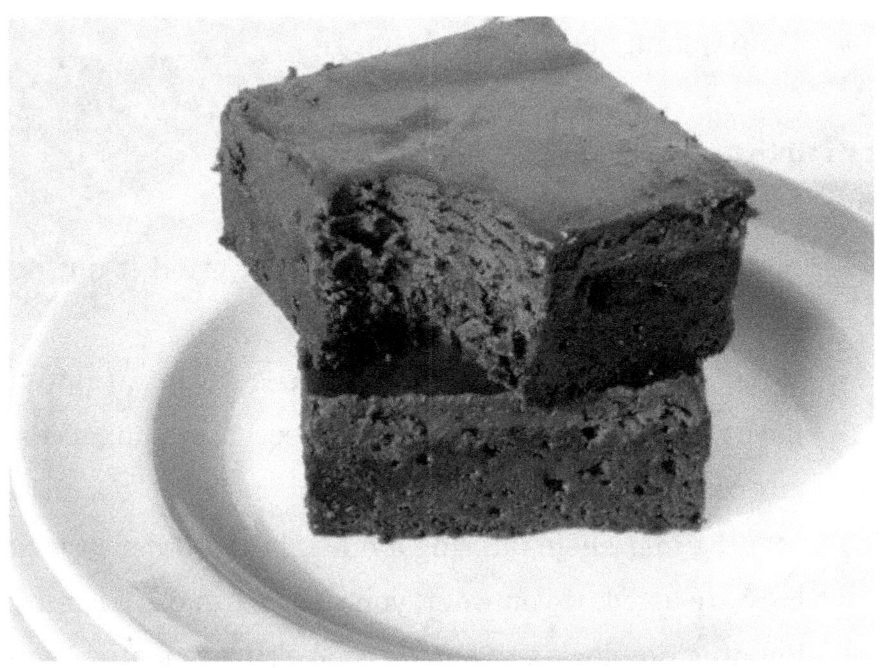

Ingredients

- Dough1 cup ground golden flaxseed or with already ground
- 4 eggs
- 1/2 cup avocado oil or any oil
- 1/2 cup granulated sweetener (maple sugar erythritol, login to, coconut sugar).
- 1/4 cup coconut flour
- 2 teaspoons vanilla
- 2 teaspoons cinnamon
- 1 teaspoon juice

- 1/2 teaspoon soda

- pinch full sea salt

- 1 cup walnut peel (leave out fine)

Instructions

- Preheat oven to 325 * F.

- If starting with whole golden flaxseed, grind it during a coffee mill, then measure 1 cup.

- Note: I prefer to use golden flax seeds because I find the flavor sweeter than dark brown flax seeds, but flax seeds of any color will work.

- Mix the ingredients during a bowl, in the order in which they are listed. If you want, you will use an electric mixer, but after employing the mixer, make sure to feature in the nut finally.

- Bake at 325 * F for 18 to 22 minutes. I like to recommend using muffin liners to prevent sticking, plus they make muffins more "portable".

Keto Egg Cake

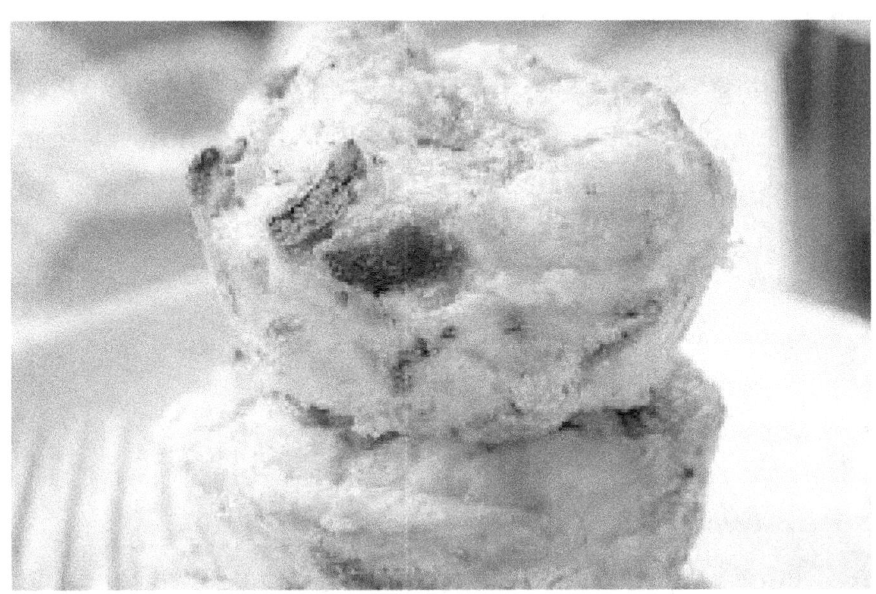

Ingredients

- 1 tbsp vegetable oil
- 8 ounces white button mushrooms chopped
- salt and freshly ground black pepper
- 10 ounces fresh spinach leaves + leaves cup water or 10 ounces frozen spinach,
- 6 eggs lightly whipped
- 6 ounces feta crumbled

Instructions

- Preheat the oven to 37575. ° F. Coat a muffin tin with nonstick cooking spray.

- To sauté the mushrooms (optional, see note): In
- a large pan over medium-high heat, heat the oil until it comes to a boil. Add the mushrooms and 1/4 teaspoon salt and cook until softened and so the mushrooms have released most of their liquid for about 5 minutes.
- Using a slotted spoon, drain the mushrooms in a bowl, leaving the remaining oil and fluid within the skillet.

To Use Fresh Spinach:

- Pour into the pan with water and sauce until tender and wilted about 10 minutes. Drain and place during a clean kitchen towel. Squeeze and rotate the towel to get rid of the maximum amount of liquid as possible.
- To use frozen spinach (melted):
- Sauté in a pan until heated through, about 5 minutes. Drain and place during a clean kitchen towel. Squeeze and rotate the towel to get rid of the maximum amount of liquid as possible.
- To make egg muffins:
- Add spinach to the bowl with the mushrooms. Stir in eggs, cheese, 1/2 teaspoon salt and 1/4 teaspoon pepper.
- Divide the egg mixture evenly into 12 muffin cups. Bake for about 25 minutes until a toothpick is cleaned.

- Cool slightly before removing from muffin tins (egg cups should start easily). Serve hot or at temperature. Store leftovers within the refrigerator and use within 4 days.
- To freeze the muffins:
- cool and transfer in a single layer on a plate. Freeze until freezing, for a minimum of half an hour, then transfer to a freezer-safe bag. Freeze for 2 months.
- To heat the muffins:
- Microwave directly from the freezer until heated for about 1 minute.

Chapter 6: Frozen Desserts Recipes

The Homemade Sneakers

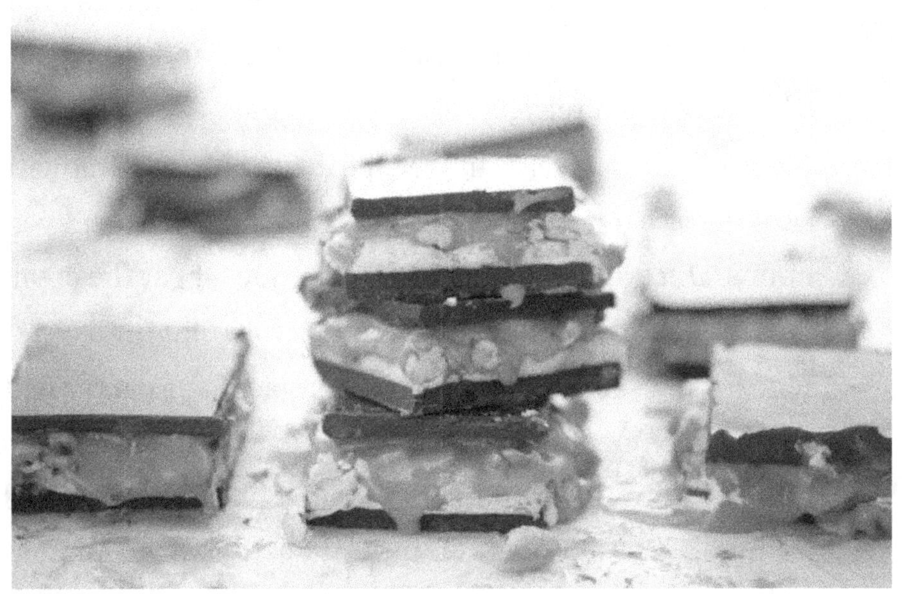

Ingredients

- 1/2 cup caramel Cato, 6 is designed with a large spoon. Butter and eight tablespoons cream
- 4 oz. (113g) cheese, temperature
- 1 1/2 cups (355mL) cream
- 1 cup (240mL) natural creamy

- 1/2 cup peanuts
- 6.5 oz (184g) 85% bittersweet chocolate or sugar-free chocolate tbsp
- 2 cups oil

Instructions

- Make caramel sauce as directed, using 6 tablespoons butter and eight tablespoons cream. Cool and keep aside (these are often refrigerated for three days ahead.) In
- the bowl of an electric mixer, beat the cheese. Gradually add the cream, scrape the bowl repeatedly to prevent lumps. Once all the cream has been added, beat the cream mixture to form stiff peaks. Carefully fold into the spread.
- Line a 9 × 9-inch square pan with 2 pieces of parchment, so the parchment hangs on each edge. Spread the mixture evenly within the bottom of the pan. Sprinkle evenly with peanuts, pressing lightly into the spreading mixture. Drizzle caramel sauce over peanuts and keep inside the freezer for 3 hours or overnight.
- Once completely frozen, use the parchment to lift the frozen dessert out of the pan and into the chopping board. Dig 24 times too. Divide the bars into 2 sets of 12 and place each assay on a parchment-lined baking sheet. Place the chocolate back inside the freezer to melt.

- Melt the chocolate with copra oil on a double-boiler or within a microwave for 30 seconds, then 10 seconds, stirring occasionally, until melted.
- Working with one sheet at a time, tap the extra chocolate, dipping each bar into the chocolate with a fork. Place back on the baking sheet. When all the bars are covered, return the baking sheet to the freezer and repeat with the opposite batch.
- Once the chocolate is completely set, move the bar to an airtight container and freeze for three months.

Chocolate Chip Cookie Sandwiches

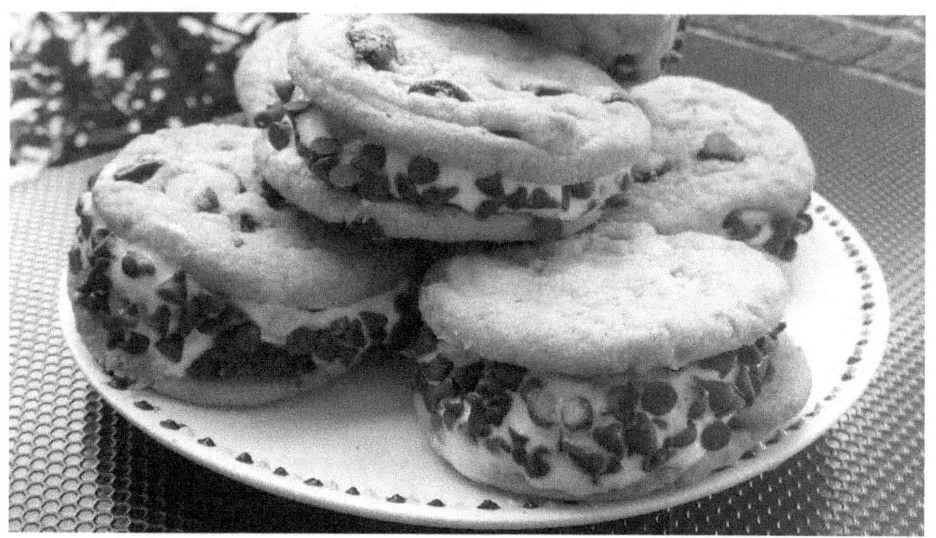

Ingredients

Cookie Dough:

- 4 tablespoons butter
- 4 tablespoons cheese
- 2 cups almond flour
- 1/2 cup Trim Healthy Mama Gentle Sweet or my sweetener
- 1 tsp jaggery ***
- 1 tablespoon vanilla
- 1 cup sugar-free chocolate chips or chopped sugar-free chocolate or chocolate

Ice Cream:

- 2 cups cream

- 1 cup half milk
- 1 cup almond
- 3 egg yolks
- 1/2 cup Trim Healthy Mama Gentle Sweet or myself Tin
- 1 teaspoon vanilla
- 1 tbsp glycerin
- 1 cup sugar-free chocolate chips optional

Instructions

- In an 8x8 square baking pan with a line with parchment paper or foil.
- Beat butter, cheese, and sweetener with a mixer. Add almond flour, sweetener, vanilla, and jaggery within. Mix well Stir within the chocolate chips. Place half the cookie dough in the bottom of the pan and spread it gently. Cover with another layer of parchment or foil. Spread the remainder of the dough on the second layer. (The pictures here help with this). Keep it inside the freezer.
- Meanwhile, make frozen dessert. Combine all frozen dessert ingredients during a blender. Blend until smooth. Pour into a frozen dessert machine and churn according to the manufacturer's instructions. If desired, add additional chocolate chips during the eleventh hour. When frozen, the confectionary firm removed the cookie dough from the freezer and removed the top layer. Pour 3/4 of the frozen

dessert on top of the rock bottom layer of cookie dough. Save the rest in another container.

- It is best not to top it with the highest cookie dough yet. You'll want to give it a touch and set. So put this and therefore separate the top layer of dough inside the freezer. After an hour or two, remove them from the freezer and top the frozen dessert with the highest layer of cookie dough.

- Freeze for another 3-4 hours. It is often when it is good that there was a touch of leftover frozen dessert. It is so difficult to be patient. Eat a touch of extra while waiting.

- Remove from the freezer and dig squares with a pointed knife. Wrap individually with wrapping to store.

Keto Chocolate Covered Barsplace

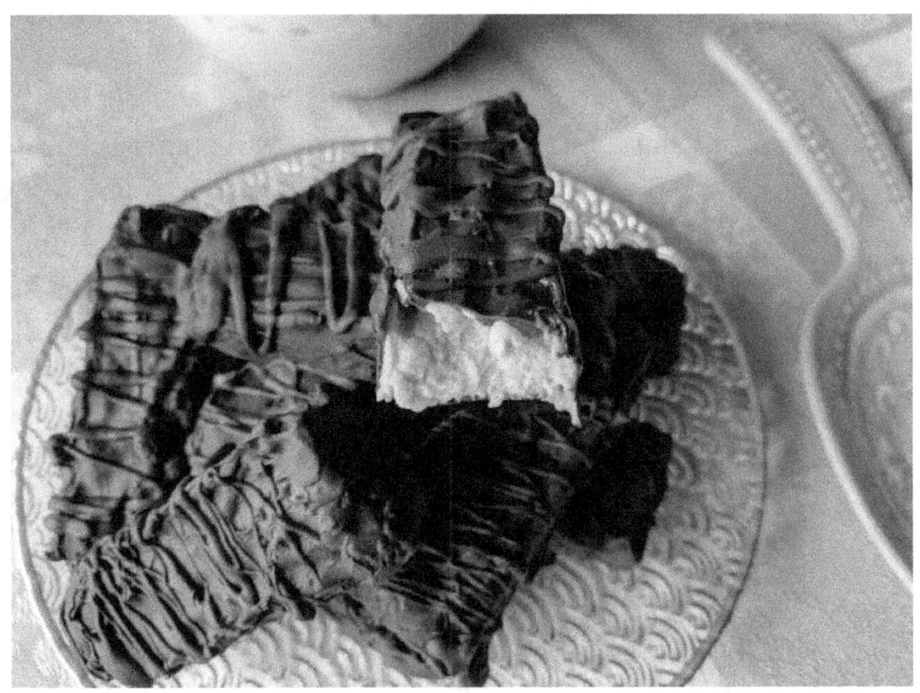

Ingredients

- 1 cup Heavy Light Whipping Cream
- 1 cup Almond milk
- 2/3 s. Natural Peanut Butter
- 3T. xylitol (or more, to taste)
- 1 t. Vegetable Glycerin (optional)
- 1 tsp. Vanilla
- 1/16 teaspoon. THM Pure Stevia Extract Powder (or any concentrated stevia powder)
- ¾ tsp. xanthan gum

- Refined copra oil

- 2 oz. unsweetened baker's chocolate

- Chopped cocoa butter pieces

- 3 c / tsp. THM Super Sweet Blend (or more, to taste) (or find out what the ratio of your favorite sweetener is here)

- Dash Salt

Instructions

Ice Cream:

- Blend frozen confectionery ingredients for 30 seconds, blending fine Mix the xanthan gum first. Therefore, it is not to collide.

- Churn the frozen sweetmeat mixture during 1 t - qt. Chop frozen sweets according to the manufacturer's instructions.

- Spread the prepared frozen dessert in a foil-row 9 "x13" pan, cover, and freeze

- Press the frozen dessert into 15 bars with a knife, when it is partially frozen, continue to solidify until firm.

Dipping Chocolate:

- Melt all ingredients together within the microwave or during a double saucepan, frequently stirring so the chocolate does not burn.

- Let the melted mixture cool down a touch before dipping your frozen dessert bar so that it does not melt the frozen dessert.

- I need frozen dessert bars on the outside of their pan (foil helps with this) and dip them one at a time within the chocolate mixture, dip one side, flip to dip in the opposite direction, then hold. Flipping again the highest with an extra coat.

- Store frozen dessert bars during a sealed freezer container.

- Frozen confectionery bars are straight out of the freezer. Still, I prefer to thaw them for 5–10 minutes before eating for a creamier texture.

Keto Froze Confectionery Cake

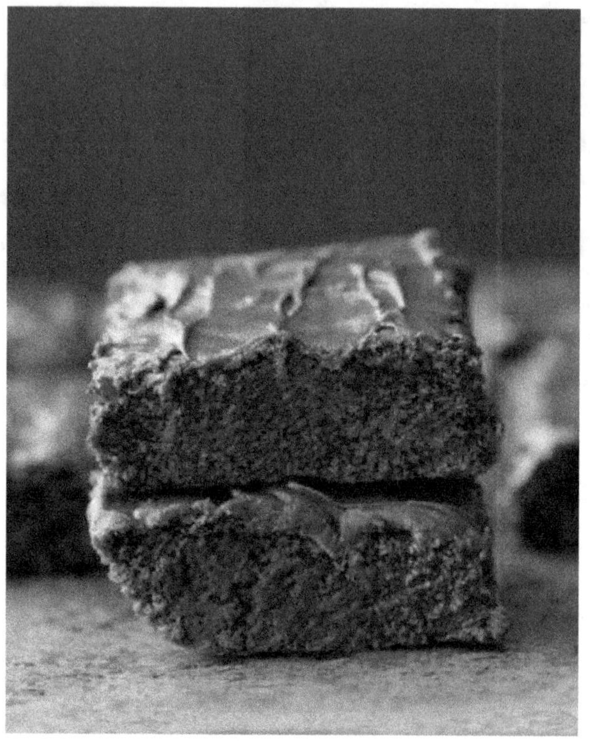

Ingredients

Cake:

- 1 cup almond flour
- 1/4 cup sweet sweetener
- 1/4 cup chocolate
- 1 1/2 tsp lever
- 1/4 tsp salt
- 2 large eggs, temperature
- 1/2 cup butter, melted.

- 1/2 teaspoon vanilla
- 2 to 4 cold coffee or water

Ice Cream:

- 2 cups heavy light cream whipping cup bacha
- Tablespoon 1/2sweet split (or allulose or xylitol) sweetened sweetener spoon Aniston 1/2 tbsp xanthan
- 6 tbsp powder
- 3 tbsp butter
- 1 cup chopped fresh strawberries
- 12 ounces of cheese soft
- Chocolate Glaze:
- 1/2 cup Heavy Light Whipping cream
- 2 ounces Anzac chocolate and cuts chickpea
- chocolate 1/4 cup powdered sweetener
- 1/2 T Pun vanilla

Instructions

- Cake Greece to preheat and 9 325F oven inch Springform pan well. Rock bottom and parchment oil lined with parchment paper.
- In a medium bowl, whisk together almond flour, chocolate, yeast, and salt. Add eggs, melted butter, and vanilla and stir to mix. Add coffee or water 1 tbsp at a time

until spreading consistency is achieved. The solution should not be touched.

- Spread the batter evenly within the prepared baking pan and remain firm for half an hour or just to the touch. Remove and let cool completely. Once it cools completely, runs a pointed knife over the sides of the pan and loosen the edges. Then tighten the edges (this is simply to make sure the cake does not stick to the pan sides after freezing).

Ice Cream:

- In a large, heavy saucepan during medium heat, mix light whipping cream with 6 tablespoons of Boca Sweet and each powder. Bring back to just one boil, then reduce the heat and simmer gently for half an hour. Watch carefully as you would like it to boil but still do not boil. There should be little bubbles along the sides throughout.

- Remove from heat and whisk within the butter until melted. Sprinkle xanthan gum and whisk on the surface to harden it. Let the temperature cool down, about 20 minutes.

- Meanwhile, place the strawberries during a blender with the remaining 2 tablespoons of Bacha Sweet. Puree and set aside.

- In a large kitchen appliance, combine cheese and, therefore, cream mixture. Beat until very smooth. Taste for sweetness and if you want it a touch sweeter, add more powder. Add more vanilla if desired.

- Spread this mixture on about 2/3 evenly cooled cakes.
- Add strawberry puree to the remaining mixture within the kitchen appliance and mix to blend, scraping down the sides of the kitchen appliance to ensure that it is all in the mixture. Again, taste for sweetness.
- Spread this mixture on top of the vanilla within the pan, smoothening the most. Freeze until firm, about 6 hours.

Chocolate Glaze:
- In a small saucepan over medium heat, bring the cream to just a boil. Remove from heat and add the chopped chocolate. Let sit for two minutes, then whisk within the sweetener and vanilla.
- Let it thicken for 5 minutes, then pour over the top of the cake and let the edges drip down. On frozen cakes, it will harden quickly.
- To serve, preheat a pointed knife or heat the gas range (this is what I do!). Slice straight down, making sure to cut through the rock bottom cake layer. Work a spatula under the cake but on parchment paper.

Peanut Butter and Jelly Sandwich

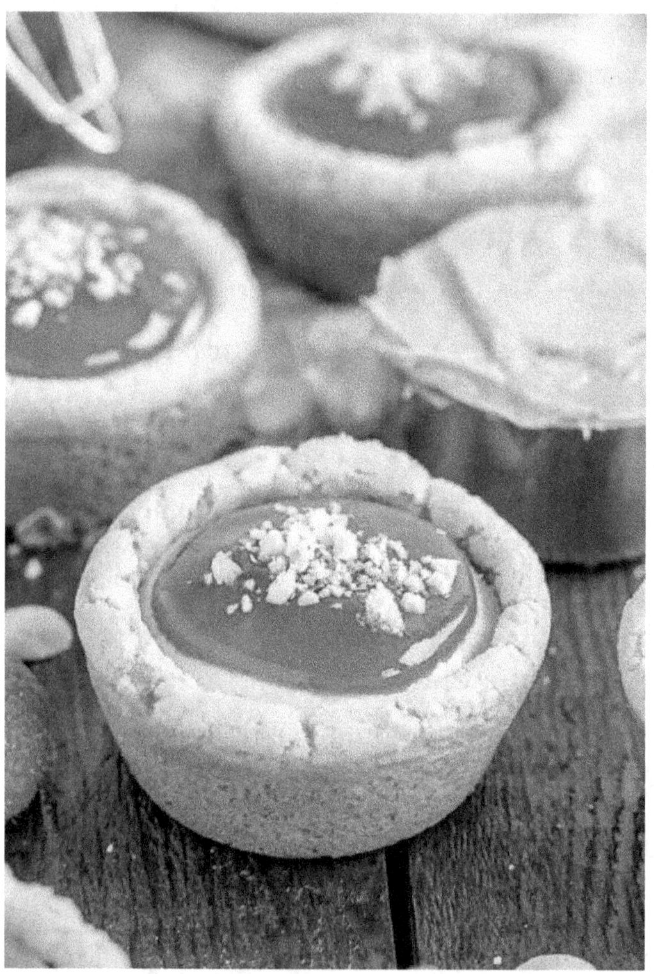

Ingredients

Peanut Butter Cookies:

- Cut the Keto Watt Spread Bars 2 times in half, see the notes. If the

- mixed berry jam

- is out of 1/2 cup of the mixed berries, if they freeze, you can hear them for 15 seconds. Want to during microwave

Juice:

- 1 tablespoon chorizo on rest syrup caramel

Peanut Butter Frozen Dessert:

- 1 cup cream
- 1/4 cup powder monk fruit erythritol
- 1 tbsp choc zero upright caramel or 1 tsp vanilla
- 2 tablespoons chunky salted or creamy

Instructions

Keto Watt:

- Spread Cookies Heat the oven to 350 degrees. Put the keto watt bar into balls. Place the "dough" on the baking sheet. Counting on your back over, you will need parchment to stick.
- Level the balls with a rock bottom of a glass.
- If you make a crisscross pattern on top of the cookies, with a fork.
- Bake for 8 minutes
- Remove the cookies to cool the oven.
- Berry jam

- all the ingredients in a blender cup Add. I take advantage of this, which comes with my certified refurbished Ninja Professional Alutiiq.
- Blend on puree settings

Peanut Butter Frozen Dessert:
- Put all the ingredients high-speed blender and blend for 30 seconds. The goal is to incorporate diffusion into the cream. If you skip this step, you will spread the drops in your frozen dessert. If you mix for more than 30 seconds, you will spread to the toppings (tasty, but almost what we are going for).
- Churn the mixed cream in a frozen dessert maker or add the mixed cream to a glass jar, then freeze for 3 - 4 hours, or until the frozen dessert feels like you just like it.

Homemade Raspberry Ripple Frozen Bar
(Low Carb and Sugar-Free)

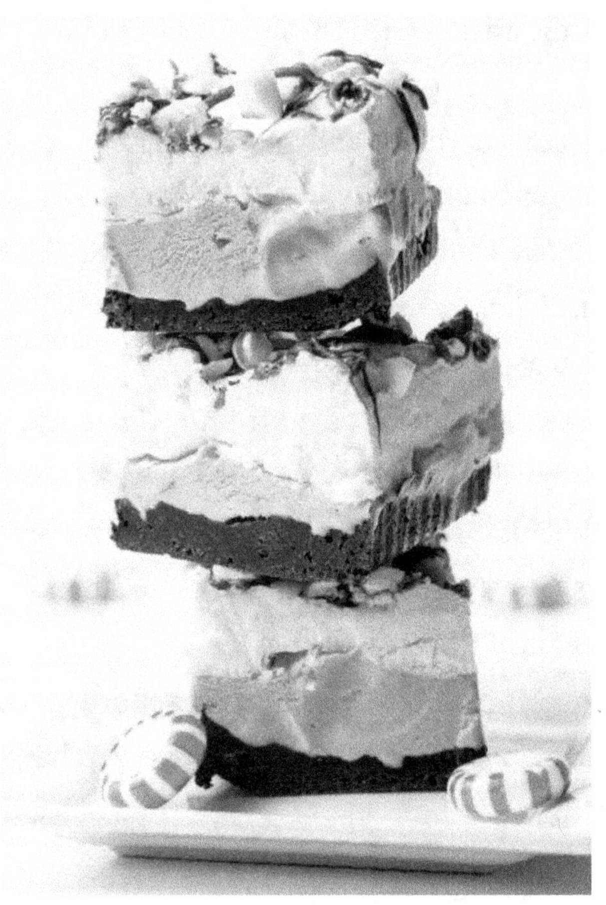

Ingredients

- 2 cups cream
- 4 cups raspberries (2 cups juice)
- 1/2 cup erythritol
- 1 tsp vanilla

Instructions

- Cook raspberries over coffee with one cup of hot water. Cook the raspberries until they release the juice.
- Press the raspberries through a sieve and squeeze out as much juice as you can most likely.
- Add 2 cups of the reserve of raspberry juice and (optional) 1 tbsp of vodka.
- Mix heavy light whipping cream with vanilla and powdered erythritol and set aside in 2 bowls. (Optional) Add 1 teaspoon of vodka.
- Pour 1/2 cup of the juice from at least one bowl of the cream bowl and vice versa 1 1/2 cups.
- Put the mixture in a popsicle mold alternately between the colors. Slowly so the mixture does not mix completely.
- Freeze until frozen.
- Remove from popsicle mold and store wrapped with a touch of parchment while in a freezer bag for up to a month.

Chapter 7: Tarts and Pies Recipes

Tarts with Low Carb Keto Berries

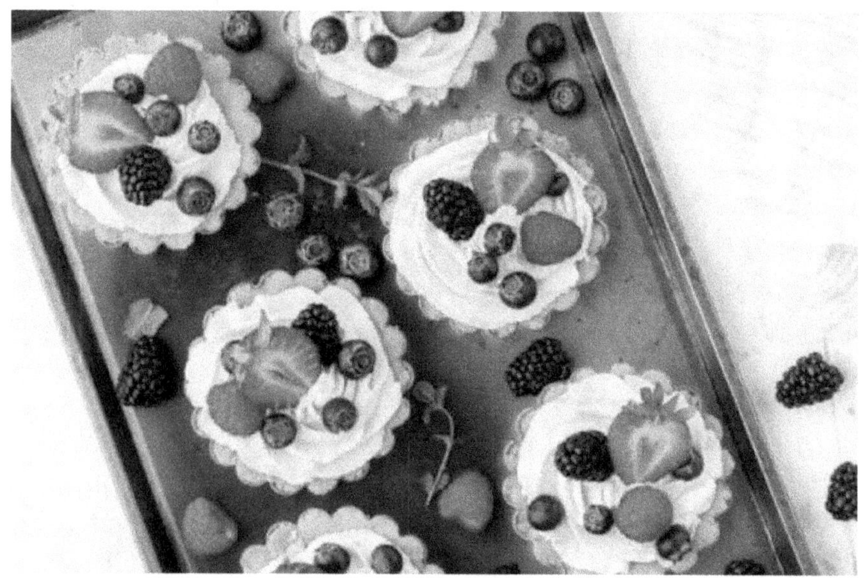

Instructions:

Tart Layer:

- Flour almonds 2 1/4 cups
- 1/4 cup powdered erythritol-I wander confectioners used
- 5 tablespoons buttermilk
- 1/4 teaspoon sea salt for

Mascarpone Cream:

- 6 oz cheese
- 2 teaspoons powdered erythritol
- 1/3 cup cream
- 1 teaspoon vanilla from Chilean Ends
- 1/4 teaspoon lemon

Decorate:

- cut 3 half strawberries
- 6 blueberries
- 6 raspberries
- 6 blackberries

Instructions

Keto Tarts:

- Oven Keto tart crust before in the six 4-inch tart sun spray copra oil or butter spray for 350 F.
- Mix almond flour, butter, salt and sweetener in a bowl. Match to include.
- Divide the dough into a six-tart pan and rock between the rock bottom and the walls. Make holes under the rock of flour, employing a fork. Bake for 8–10 minutes until golden, then remove the oven and funky completely.

Mascarpone Cream:

- Beat mascarpone and powdered sweetener with an electric mixer for two minutes at low speed. Beats at low speed, gradually add cream.
- Increase the speed and beat for 30-60 seconds, until thick. Be very careful, because now you will beat the cream and it will fall apart. The focus of low speed, temperature, mascarpone, and ton is important here! Hammer in lemon peel and vanilla.

Low Carb Lemon Cheese Flavor

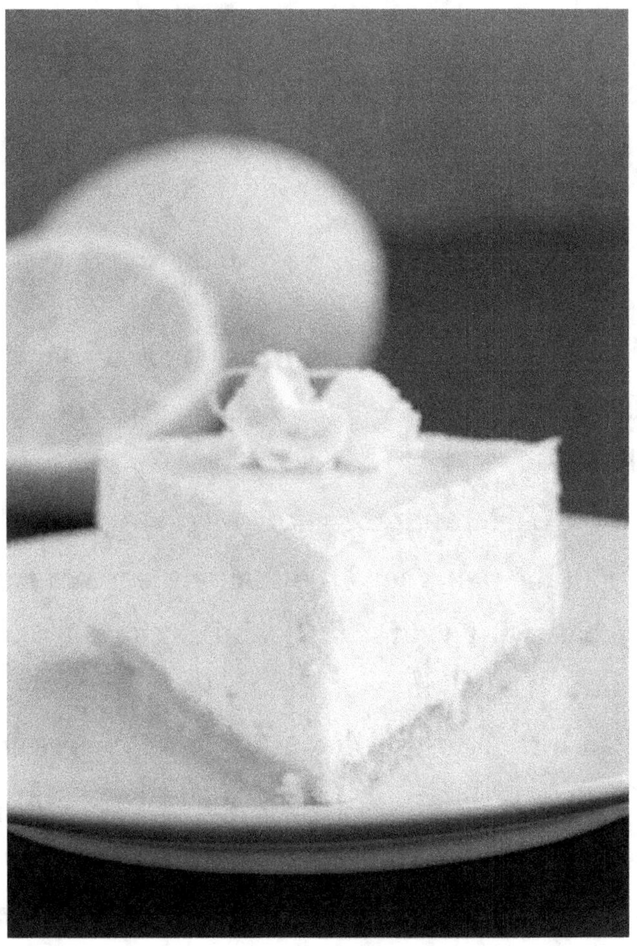

Ingredients

Lemon Cheese:

- 340 g (11.99 oz) blackberry (or other fruit)
- 1 tbsp chopped almonds
- Sprinkle and Parchment Paper

Almond Flour Pie Crust:

- 210 g (7.41 oz) Blended Almond Flour (about 1.5 cups)
- 70 g (2.47 oz) Coconut Flour (about 1/2 cup)
- 50 g (2.82 oz) powder erythritol (about in) see 4 tbsp)
- 2 eggs
- 4 tbsp cold unsalted butter (or refined coconut oil)

Instructions

- Make a recipe for lemon cheese and cool it within the fridge.
- Heat the oven to 180C / 350F.
- Keep all the pie. Knead the shell ingredients and a sphere or a ball with your hands until it forms a large bowl. Separate the ball in two. This makes 2 pies on the way.
- In your tart molds, spray some oil everywhere and Though Create Ha little round portal. Paper rock bottom so that the crust does not stick.
- Add tart mold to the balls of dough. Keep up the surround Press urn fingers with you until crust evenly in the mold. Do not spread. With a fork, gently press the dough with a knife to create small air pockets in several places.
- Add crusts to the oven and bake for a quarter of an hour. Take it out and let it cool completely before adding lemon cheese.

- After the pie shell cools, gently take it out of the mold and transfer it to the dish of your choice.

- Spread half lemon cheese on each tart and canopy with blackberries. You will then add slices of almonds everywhere and sprinkle a touch of erythritol powder on the blackberry to create that grainy sugar look.

- Be sure to eat this pie on an equal day as the lemon cheese crystallizes inside the fridge when it is exposed to air due to erythritol. I had personally eaten it within three days and so the curd was crisp to the touch not in some places but throughout the custard.

Strawberry Mascarpone Tarts

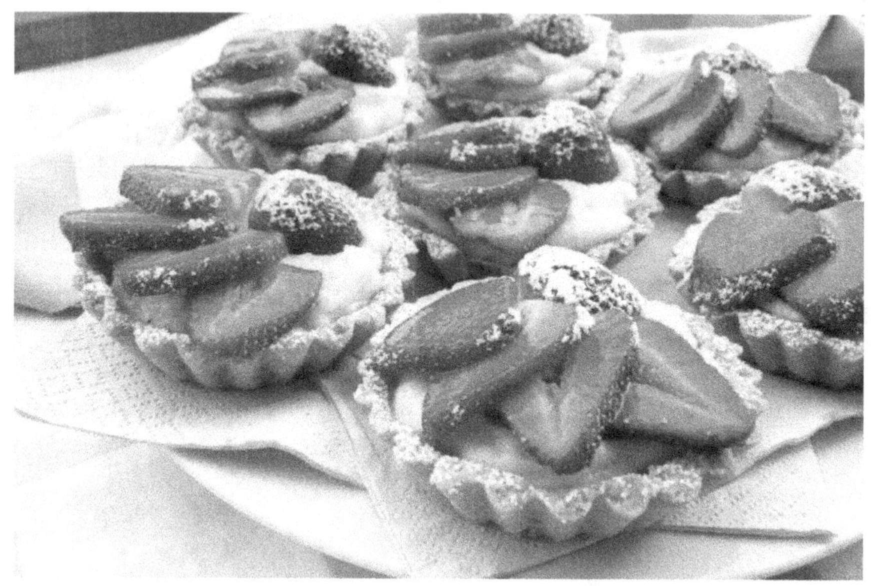

Ingredients

Coconut Base:

- 1/2 cup copra oil
- 100g / 3/4 cup plus 2 tablespoons coconut flour
- 2 eggs
- 1 tsp vanilla
- 1 tsp powdered sweetener

Mascarpone Cream:

- 250g / 8.8 Ounce / 1 very generous cup of mascarpone
- 2 eggs
- 1 tsp vanilla

- 1-2 teaspoon ground sweetener
- 200 g / 1 cup strawberry
-

Instructions

- Heat your oven to 180 C / 356 Fahrenheit.
- If using, beat your eggs with copra oil, vanilla, and sweetener of choice. I used my kitchen tools, but it would be through a stick blender.
- Add in coconut flour and mix.
- Your dough should be soft but not too sticky. If necessary, add a touch more coconut flour to urge proper consistency. You will also stick the dough inside the fridge for 10 minutes to cool it - this can make it easier to roll out.
- Now you have 2 options: either roll the dough between 2 sheets of baking paper. Or press it directly into a pie form that you simply lined with parchment paper or pounded well with copra oil.
- Bake for about 10 minutes or until lightly browned on the sides.
- Now make your filling: Separate the eggs and beat the egg white during a cleanup!! And dry!! Porcelain or metal bowl with a handheld or electric metal whisk. As you will see within the photo, I used an old-fashioned whisk and about 2 minutes of muscle power. You will roll in the grass too! Until hard peaks stop forming, do not believe in mixing

mascarpone and, therefore, egg yolk, then vanilla and sweetener.

- Gently fold the hardened egg whites within.
- Once the tart base has cooled, add the mascarpone mixture.
- Refrigerate within the fridge until served (at least 1/2 hour).
- Just before serving, add strawberries - sliced, halved, or fully, however you favor.

Keto Chocolate Tart

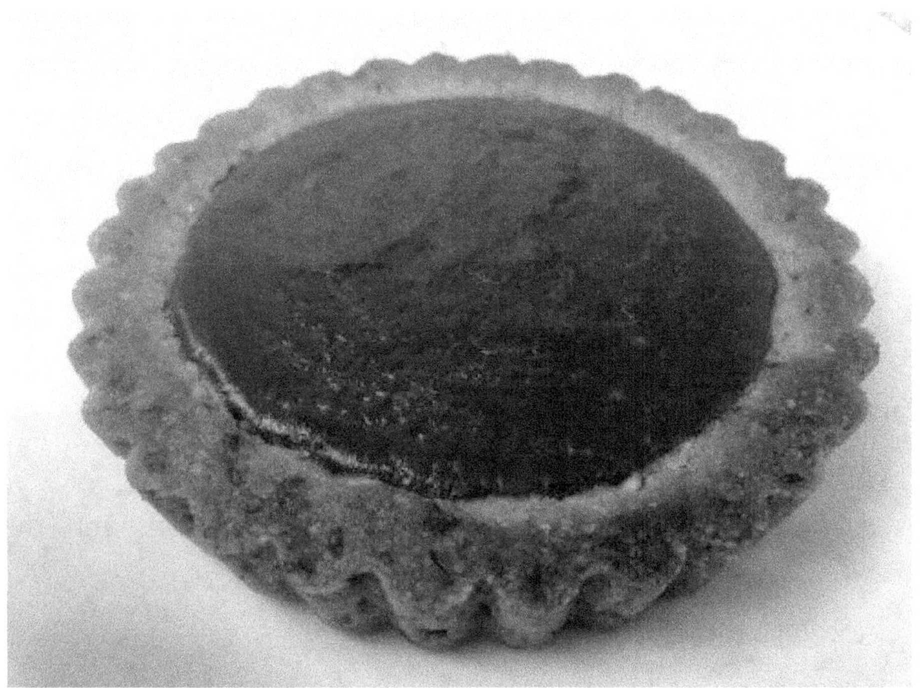

Ingredients

Crust:

- 1 Cup Almond Flour Wet Unarmed
- 6 tbsp Melted Butter

Tart:

- 1 Heavy Cup Heavy Light Whipping Cream
- 9 oz Unwanted Chocolate (Chopped or Broken into)
- 1 tsp Vanilla
- 2 Eggs (room temperature)

- ½ tsp salt
- 1 cup Sweater, Infers N's

Glaze:

- 2 Oz Awakened chocolate
- 1/4 cup Silver, Infers N's
- 1/2 cup light Whipping cream
- 2 tablespoons sour cream

Instructions

- Heat until between 325 ° F oven with a rack.
- Stir all the ingredients together and press evenly into the bottom of the tart pan.
- Bake on the firm for about 10 minutes.
- Cool on a wire rack for 15 to twenty minutes.
- Increase the oven temperature to 350 degrees.
- Bring cream to a boil, then add chopped chocolate during a bowl and let stand for 5 minutes. Stir gently until smooth.
- In a separate bowl, stir together vanilla, eggs, salt and curly, then melted chocolate.
- Pour the filling into the cold crust. Bake until the filling is about, and the center is slightly wobbly - about 15 to twenty minutes.
- Cool completely in a pan on a rack for about 1 hour. The center will still be set as tart cold.

Glaze:

- In a saucepan over medium-low heat, add chocolate, swears, cream, and sour cream.
- Stir the mixture continuously and roast the sugarcane till it becomes smooth and hot.
- Pour over the cold tart and tilt it slightly to help the glaze to cover the tart fully.
- Let cool for an hour and add swipe light whipping cream or raspberry sauce on top.

Note: If you make it the day before an occasion or party, set it in the refrigerator overnight. Apply glaze for an hour or two before serving. The glaze will lose a lot of shine within the fridge.

Coconut Flour Pie Shell

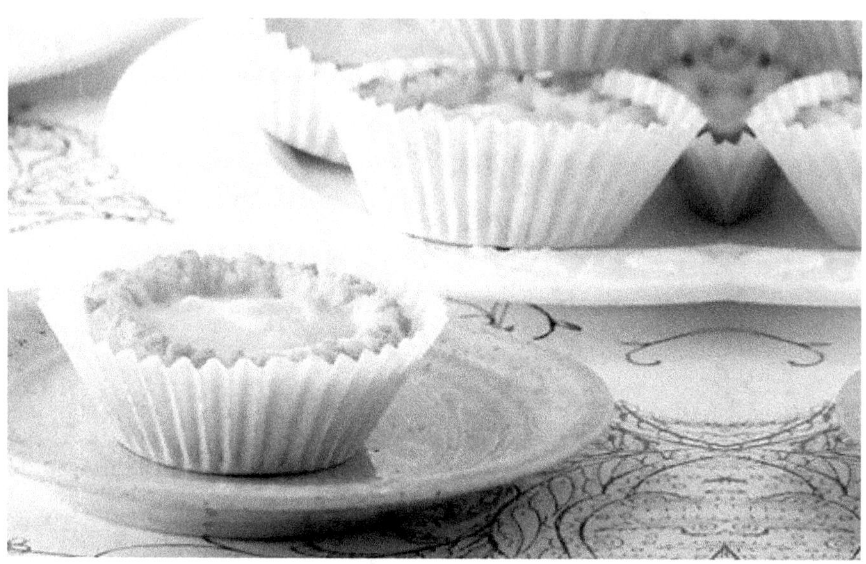

Ingredients

- 3/4 cup coconut flour
- 2 eggs
- 1/3 cup extra virgin coconut oil
- 1/4 teaspoon salt or 1 tbsp powder A sweet pie for sweetener
- Sweet pie shell
- 2 tbsp erythritol
- 1 teaspoon ground cinnamon
- 1 teaspoon ground ginger
- 1 teaspoon rind of lemon
- pie shell

- 1 teaspoon salt

- 1teaspoon garlic powder

Instructions

- Keep reading for full detailed instructions.

- Preheat oven fan forced 180C (350 F) to

- a 24 cm (9 in) pie pan with butter or copra oil. I like to recommend a nonstick removable bottom pan; this will make the molding process easier. Otherwise, glass or ceramic pan also works, but you will need to serve the pie and pan there.

- In a large bowl (or a kitchen appliance with an S blade attachment), coconut flour, beaten eggs (at room temperature), melted copra oil (not hot, lukewarm, hot oil burnt eggs!) And salt (or sweetener Count) add. On making your savory pie or sweet pie).

- Mix with a spoon (or process on medium speed until it becomes a thick dough). The dough is initially wet and dries as you go. After 30 seconds, use your hands to knead the dough, it should not take much more than 90 seconds to get ready to make the dough ball. If you use a kitchen appliance, it will make a piece of dough after 30–45 seconds. Stop the food processor, gather the pieces together with your hands in a ball.

Press Into Method:

- If you do not wish to roll the dough, just place the dough ball within the center of the dough pan. Press with your hand to flatten the ball. It will slowly be re-created; this is what you want to possess with an amazing shortbread coconut pie shell. Use your finger to spread and press the dough evenly everywhere in the pan and press the dough to stay in the pan until it forms a sizzling smooth crust.

- Use the back of a spoon to press the dough into the pan and smooth the surface. The more you press it while serving, the higher it will be.

Rolling Method:

- Place the dough on a bit of parchment paper, press another piece of parchment paper on top. Yes, you do not need to cool the dough at this level!

- Roll out the dough, thick as a regular pie shell. Refrigerate the rolled dough for 10 minutes on a flat board. This will harden the dough slightly and make it easier to roll over the pan.

- Remove the highest layer of parchment paper and flip the crust on the pan.

- Remove the last parchment paper layer and press the dough into the center to go inside the pan. It will be fixed. Gather the dough pieces to fill the hole and press them with your fingers to stay. Use a spoon to smooth the surface.

- Pre-baking prick. Avoid over-pressing the dough at pan boundaries or it becomes difficult to serve slices without breaking.

- Bake pre-quarter-hour at 350 C so that the top side of the border is too brown to add brown foil.

- Remove from the oven, add the sweet or savory filling of your choice such as zest stuffing, pumpkin filling.

- Return to the oven for about 40-50 minutes for a pie or 30-40 minutes for a quickie.

- If you use a removable bottom pan, then you will be ready to unmold your pie after it has cooled within the pan at temperature for 3 hours. For ceramic and glass pans, do not serve precious and serve directly from the pan.

Chocolate Paleo and Keto French Silk Pie

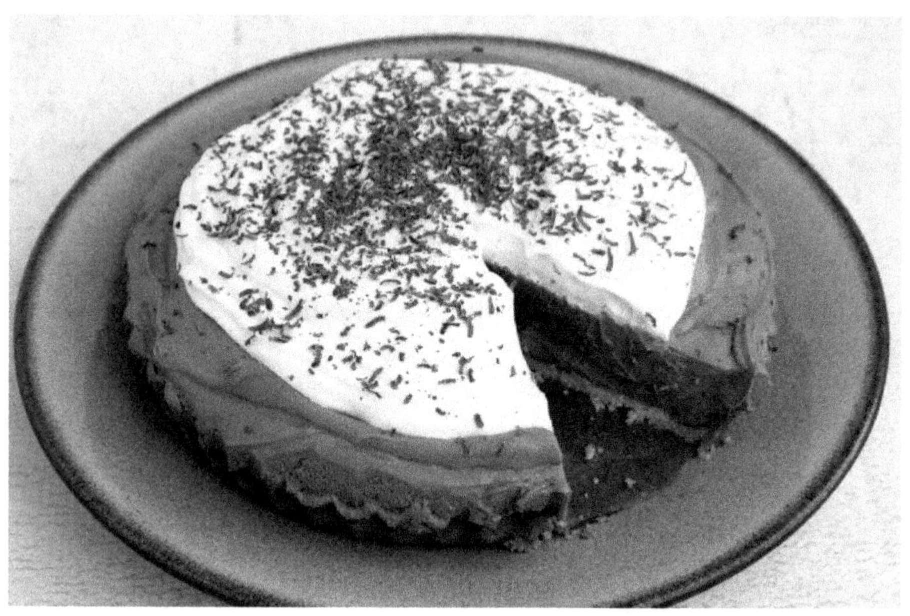

Ingredients

Keto 'Oreo' Layer:

- 25 grams of Almond Flour
- 2 tablespoons chocolate
- 2-3 tablespoons powdered erythritol or powder allulose/xylitol
- 1/8 teaspoon instant coffee
- pinch Kosher salt
- 2 -3 tablespoons Melted grass-free unsalted butter or ghee/coconut oil, as needed, 80ml

Keto Chocolate Silk Pie:

- Full-fat coconut milk
- 5-10 g chocolate or raw cocoa (to taste) for
- 2-3 tablespoons Powder earth Is mixed in Idol. Powdered allulose / xylitol, taste,
- about half a medium to about 50 grams avocado
- 1/2 teaspoon vanilla
- 1/4 teaspoon instant coffee optional
- 1/8 teaspoon kosher salt

Instructions

Keto 'Oreo' Layer:

- For layer lightly while the almond flour toast completely, dry pan or pan on medium heat until golden and fragrant (2-4 minutes).
- This is often important taste-wise, so don't skip it!
- Transfer the almond flour to a small bowl (or go straight for the serving glass), and mix in cocoa, sweetener, coffee (optional) and salt. Add to the butter, mix until well combined. When you make the cheesecake, press into a (4 1/2-inch / 12 cm) pie dish or serving glass and refrigerate.

Keto Chocolate Silk Pie:

- The thickness of your silk pie will be found largely in your coconut milk. So, use the solid portion for more 'set' pie,

- or keep it briefly to include all the milk for mild consistency (our preference!) During a water bath.

- Add all the filling ingredients to a filling blender-friendly container and mix until cream is smooth. Alternatively, place a kitchen appliance and all ingredients during mixing. Taste for sweetness and spice and adjust according to more sweetener or salt.

- Transfer to a prepared pie dish or serving glass and chill until completely set. You will always keep it in the freezer for a quarter of an hour. This chocolate silk pie stays well inside the fridge for a few days.

- If you are imagining: Garnish freshly with toppings.

No-Bake Keto Pie

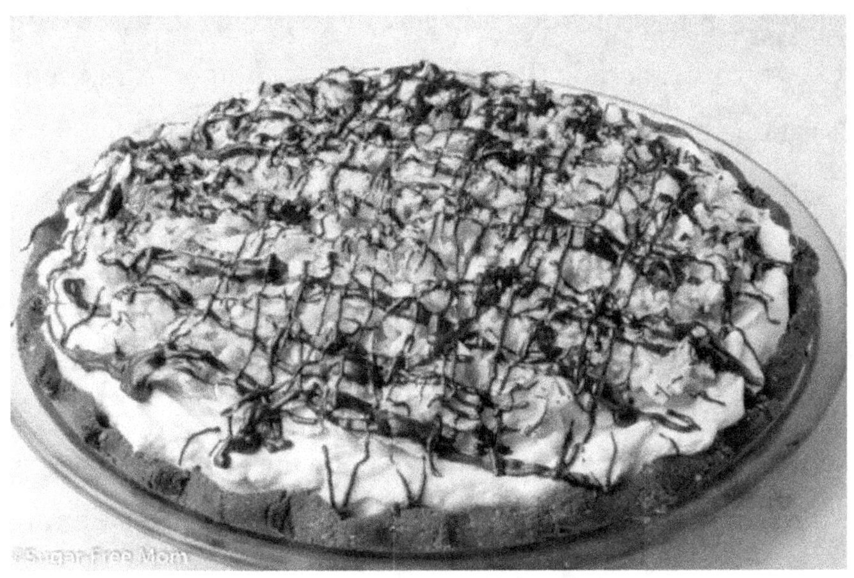

Ingredients

- 3 tablespoons copra oil, ghee or butter,
- 1/2 cup coconut milk
- 2 tablespoons collage Latin
- 15 ounces steamed pumpkin or BPA-free canned pumpkin puree
- 3 tablespoons cinnamon tablespoons.
- 2 Vanilla
- Salt Ki Chuka
- *Optional*: 1/8 teaspoon ground cloves or 1/8 teaspoon cardamom

Instructions

- Prepare before the crust. During the kitchen appliance or high-power blender, add coconut and blitz until it becomes very fine. Scrape the sides of your container as needed.

- Add the remaining crust ingredients to your blender and blend again until well incorporated.

- Line a 9-inch cake pan or pie plate with parchment and mix the mixture with your hands and then insist on packing it as much as possible with the back of a spoon. Keep your freezer in line.

- Prepare the keto pie filling. During a small bowl, mix collage Latin and water and keep it to thaw for a minute or two.

- In a saucepan over low heat, add coconut milk and so on to the collagen collage Latin and mix until dissolved and smooth.

- Add the coconut mixture to a blender along with the remaining ingredients and blend again until smooth.

- Remove your pan from the freezer and top it with the pie base. Refrigerate until set (or freeze if you are short on time).

- Serve cold with Keto Vanilla Frozen Dessert or Whipped Coconut Milk.

Gluten-Free Shulk Paleo and Keto Lime Pie

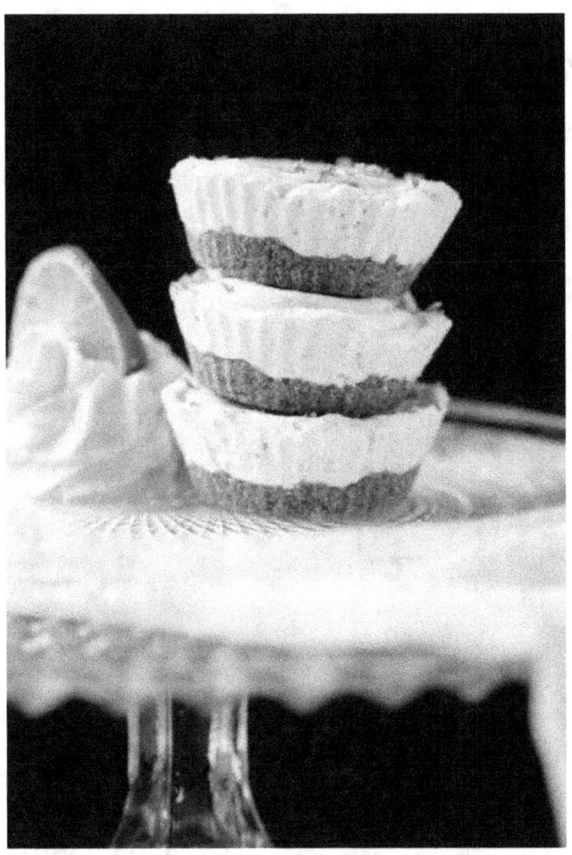

Ingredients

Keto Cracker Crust:

- 192 grams almond flour or (both work great!)
- 1 / 4-1 / 2 cup powdered xylitol or choice of sweetener, to taste
- Cinnamon 1 teaspoon
- 1/4 teaspoon Kosher salt

- 56 g unsalted grass-fed butter or ghee/coconut oil, as required,

Keto Lime Pie:

- 400 g avocado
- 250 g coconut milk cold
- 2 tbsp Fresh grated chum Zest
- was 80. Swaddle fresh lemon juice crust
- 1 / 3-1 / 2 cup powdered xylitol or choice, taste
- Swarna for 1 / 4-1 / 2 teaspoon kosher salt

Instructions

Keto Cracker Crust:

- Tostada a pan or almond flour pan Duranleau Overheat, until completely golden and fragrant (2–4 minutes). This is often important taste-wise, so don't skip it!
- Transfer the almond flour to a medium bowl and mix in the sweetener, cinnamon, and salt. Add to the butter, mix until well combined, and press into an 8 or 9-inch pie dish. Allow the pie to return to temperature and freeze during filling.

Keto Lime Pie:

- Blend all the filling ingredients (starting with a low volume) using an immersion blender (or high-speed blender) until creamy smooth. Taste for sweetness, touch and spice and adjust accordingly. Key limes may vary tones in taste, so start with a small amount and increase the flavor (keep in mind that flavor will develop when chilling).

- Spread the lime filling on the graham crust-lined pie and preferably refrigerate overnight (lime kick gets a lot better!). But if during pickle, you will keep it in the freezer for about an hour.
- Keep in the fridge for 3-4 days, and frozen for a month or two.

Nutella Pie

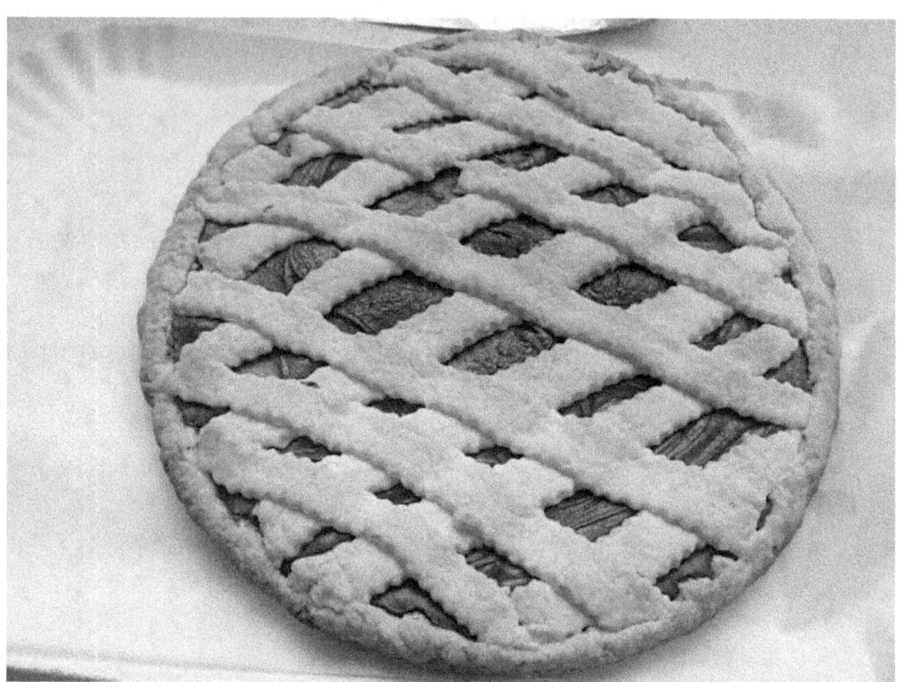

Ingredients

Crust:

- 1 1/2 cups almond flour
- 3 Tbs copra oil
- 2 1/2 teaspoons water
- 1 Parochializing
- pure stevia powder Kadesh-Yasir with 1 Karachi water instead of
- pink salt Pinch

"Nutella" Filling:

- 1 1/2 cups roasted hazelnuts - (1/4 cup for garnish)
- 1 13.6 oz Coconut Milk - Solid Cream only
- 1 3 oz Bar Bit wort Chocolate -of sugar-free pudina for keto
-
- 1 step1 teaspoon vanilla
- pinch + 1 tbsp coconut milk - or 1 Karachi Syrup, Warne for
- pink NM Kee Chuka is whipped Marilu- Garnish Lia

Instructions

- Preheat Oven to 350 degrees. A 7 "springform pan with parchment
- dry ingredients together during a bowl (flour, salt, and stevia, if used).
- paper Stir Mix in a small bowl, shake flax and water together and stir to thicken. Put aside. Melt the hemp mixture and melt the copra. Pour oil on the dry ingredients and blend well.
- Press the dough firmly into the pan. Brush the fork everywhere with a fork.
- About 15 minutes To. Firm for 15 minutes and light golden to be. A place to the cold.

Filling:

- Place the fried jackfruit in kitchen appliances. And blend until liquefied (see note
- Aside from below) Scrub and melted add the chocolate and salt. Mixture well.
- remove the into a boletates coconut milk. vanilla, 1 leftover from tbsp coconut milk (Cain) and add a pinch Stevia (or. 1 b Ha tablespoons maple syrup)
- light and thrive to whip cream with a hand mixer for 30-60 seconds.
- Leave a couple of pairs on the turn (the top gently chocolate-hazelnut mixture, if you wish So) Taste and if a touch adds more sweetener. Need.
- Pour the crust over the filling. Scoop walnuts and vortex on the remainder.
- Freeze for 1-2 hours until set. Garnish with whipped coconut milk (see notes) and chopped hazelnuts.
- Enjoy it!

Gluten-Free Keto Cocoa Pie

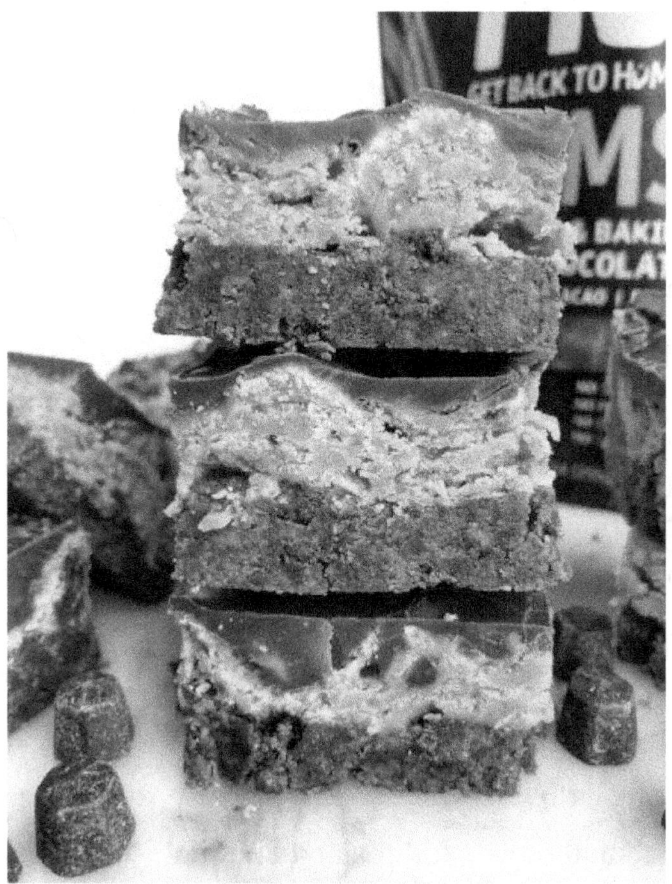

Ingredients

- 32 grams of almond flour
- 8 grams of coconut flour
- 1 tablespoon golden flaxseed meal
- 1/4 teaspoon lever
- 1/8 teaspoon kosher salt

- 42 grams grass-butter or coconut butter,

- 2-3 large Spoon LaMotte. Preferred Sweetener (we use 2TBS)

- 1/4 teaspoon vanilla

- 30g Lily Sweet Prickly Chocolate Bar Flaky (or chips)

- 20g Pecans Flaky

Instructions

- Flakey Garnish dry pan light almond flour toast or pan over medium heat, Until completely golden and fragrant (2–4 minutes). Transfer to a plate and allow to cool completely. This is often important taste-wise, so don't skip it!

- Prepare a little pie plate (about 4 inches / 11 cm diameter) or ramekin. The cookie tends to stay, so if you are not eating it directly from the dish, grease, and butter (or line).

- In a small bowl, add toasted almond flour, coconut flour, flaxseed, leaven, and salt. Keep aside until fully combined.

- Cream butter with sweetener during a medium bowl with an electric mixer until light and fluffy, scraping the edges and bottom for 3-4 minutes. Add to the vanilla and mix until fully incorporated.

- With your mixer on low, add half of your flour mixture — mixing until just incorporated. Mix within the rest.

- Fold in chocolate and pecan bits. Press into the prepared baking dish and chill within the freezer for 20 minutes.

- Preheat the oven to 350 ° F / 180 ° C, while the cookie pie is inside the freezer. Bake for 15-18 minutes until it just starts to brown.

- Let it come in line for quarter-hours before serving. Be happy to spoon it hot (right away from the dish!) With a generous scoop of our (not churned and luscious!) Vanilla frozen dessert. Alternatively, allow it to cool completely for a cookie that is slightly crisp with the edges. Store in an airtight container for 3 days (if any remaining!).

Low Carb Keto Chocolate Pie

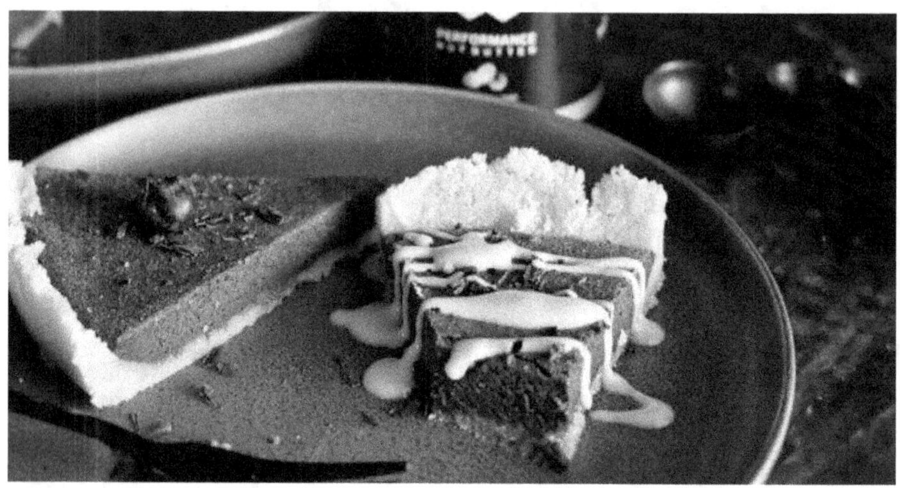

Ingredients

- Grain-free, Paleo Pie Shell
- 2 cups (260 grams) ground almonds
- m teaspoon Himalayan halite legible
- 2 teaspoons or copra oil
- 1 egg
- Chocolate
- 6 tablespoons copra oil, melted
- 3 oz. unsweetened bittersweet chocolate squares (dairy-free), melted)
- 3 eggs
- 1 cup finely chopped zucchini (255 grams freshly sliced, 195 grams. once the liquid has run out of the liquid, Hua

- 1 ml teaspoon pure vanilla

- east spoon alcohol-free Stevia

- 150 grams raw pecan halves, melted

Instructions

- Preheat the oven to 350F. For a 9 "pie, lightly grease a 9-inch pie pan with copra oil. For the 3" tarts, Lightly six with copra oil 3-inch circular tart pan.

- To make the crust, mix almond flour, salt, copra oil and egg in the bowl of your kitchen appliance. Process and pulse until a ball forms with the "S" blade, about 30 seconds. Transfer to the prepared pie or tart pan. Press the dough, pressing the edges.

- Before preparing the chocolate pie filling, be sure to "take out" the zucchini. Try to do this. For this, keep the sliced zucchini on a clean cloth and squeeze lightly. I have included the measurement of wet and dry zucchini so you can see the difference.

- Melt copra oil in the bowl of your kitchen appliance or high-power blender., Bitter chocolate, eggs, zucchini, vanilla, and stevia. Process or blend on high until smooth, about 1 minute.

- Remove the bowl of the processor from the bottom and stir in 75% pecans. If a blender is employed, transfer the chocolate mixture to a clean bowl, then stir in 75% pecans.

- Pour the chocolate pie into the prepared pie or tart pan. Top with the remaining pecans.
- For the pie, bake in a preheated oven for 35–40 minutes, until the top is smooth, and the edges are golden. Once complete, allow chilling overnight.
- For the tarts, bake in a preheated oven for 18-20 minutes, until the top is smooth, and the edges are golden. Once complete, allow cooling for 1 hour before removing from the tart pan. Tarts are often consumed or refrigerated overnight.
- Serve with coconut topping. Take six 3-inch tart or one 9-inch pie.

Keto Fudge Pie

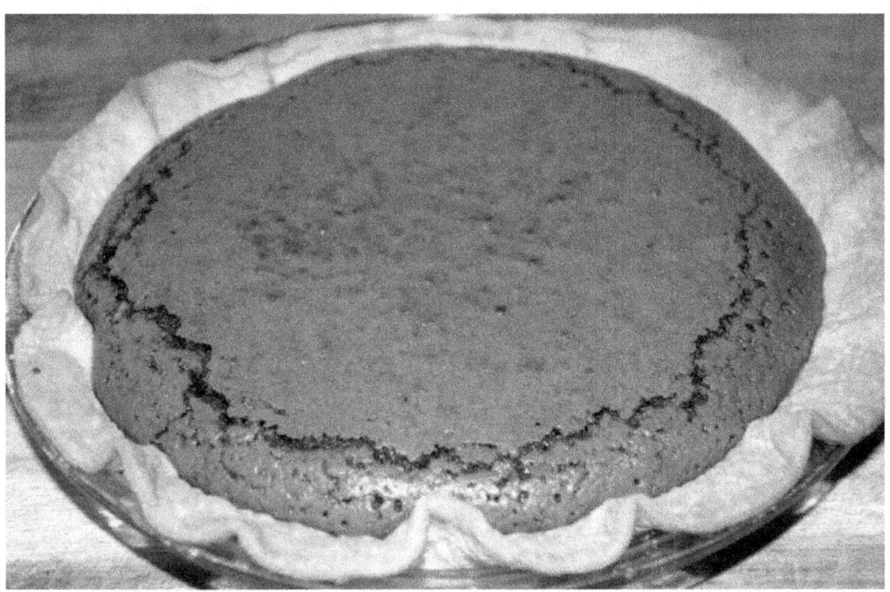

Ingredients

Crust:

- 1 cup of unsalted butter melted and cooled.
- 4 large eggs
- ½ teaspoon of sea salt
- 1 ½ cup coconut flour
- 2 Options teaspoons of sugar

Fj Byrne:

- sweet Coalesce 4 ounces
- 1/2 cup unsalted butter
- 3 eggs, temperature

- 1 cup of sugar substitute
- sea salt and 1/4 teaspoon

Instructions

Crust:

- In a large oven Preheat at 360 degrees.
- In a large bowl, mix melted butter, eggs, salt, coconut flour, and, therefore sugar.
- Just mix until the dough forms.
- Pat and press the crust into a 9-inch pie pan, allowing the crust to return the sides of the pie pan.
- Note: Wetting your hands makes it easier to pat the scab in health.
- Bake the empty pie crust for quarter-hours during a 360-degree oven.
- Cover the edges of the pie with foil to prevent it from turning brown in excess.
- Your pie shell will no longer be fully cooked as it will be baked further after filling the fud.
- Once the pie crust is baked, keep it aside and allow it to cool before frosting.

Filling Instructions:

- Melt bitter chocolate and butter during a double saucepan.
- Allow the chocolate mixture to cool completely.

- Mix eggs until thick and straw for about 3 minutes, and substitute sugar. For this use an electric mixer.
- Next, add the chocolate mixture to the egg mixture. Low-medium speed mixing until fully mixed.

Baking:
- A pre-heat 360
- Cover the edges of the pie shell with a foil. Staying on the edges of the crust due to excess browning.
- Add the Fudge to the filling in the baked pie shell.
- Bake the pie until the food is filling and the toothpick inserted comes out with moist pieces for half an hour.

Veg Keto Chocolate Almond Butter Pie

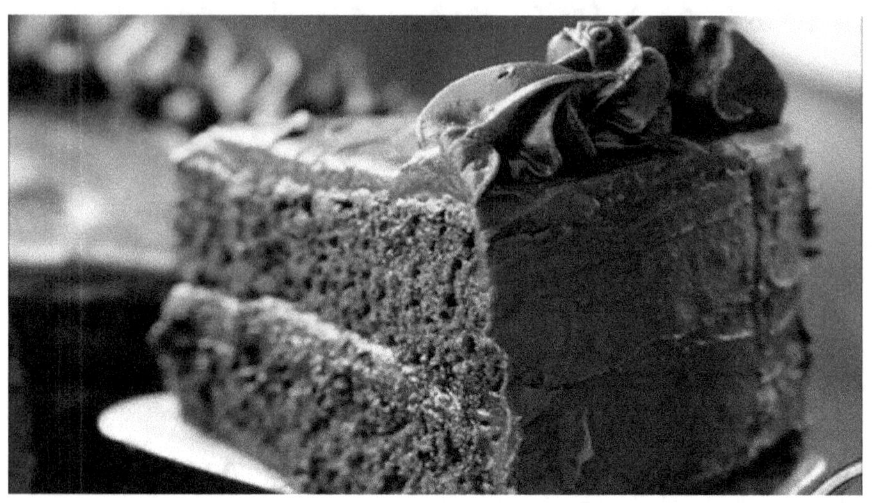

Ingredients

Crust:

- 3/4 cup (75) coconut flour
- 2 tbsp (10 g) psyllium husk
- 1/2 cup copra oil
- 1/2 cup water
- pinch of salt
- 2 ounces (30 g) Chocolate (I use Ghirardelli 100%)
- 1 can (400 ml) full fat coconut milk
- 1/4 cup copra oil
- 1 cup almond butter
- 1/4 tsp stevia (optional)

Instructions

- Preheat the oven to 350F. In a bowl, melt the water and copra oil together. Stir in psyllium husk until a type of gel forms. Next, stir in the coconut flour and salt and let sit for a minute or two, until all the liquid has been absorbed.

- Press the crust into a 9 "pie dish. Try to make the crust evenly thicker so that it remains evenly.

- Rock the bottom of the crust several times with a fork (this is called" docking ") and it helps.

- Leaving the air so the crust does not brag awkwardly) and bake for half an hour.

- While the crust is cooking, mix the remaining ingredients during a high-speed blender and whisk until they are fully combined. To make things easier, you will melt. chocolate first

- Remove them from the oven within the fridge for the 6-8 hours and chill too cool for a few minutes before falling within the crust filling until browned or freeze for 3ish hours.

- Enjoy!

Brownie Truffle Pie

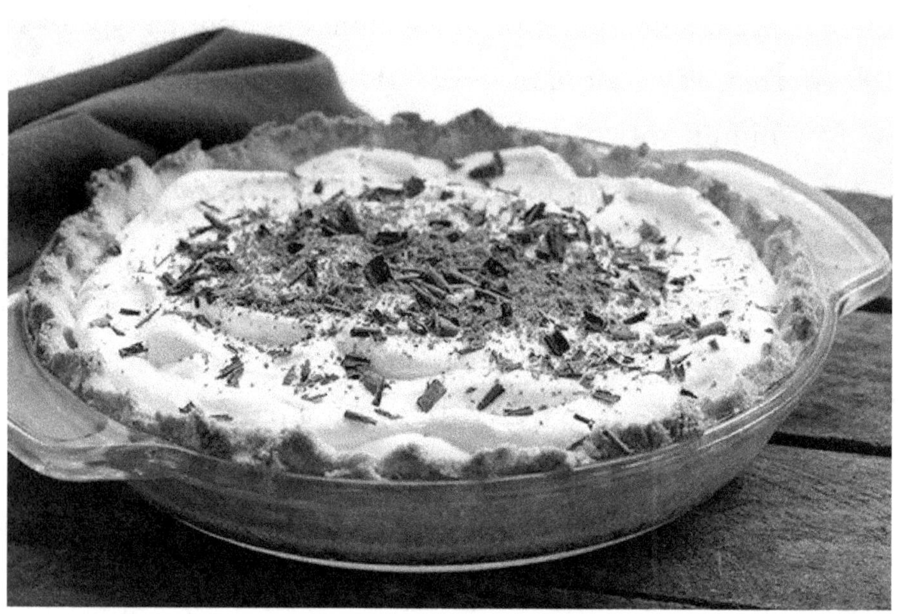

Ingredients

Crust:

- 1 1/4 cup almond flour
- 3 tablespoons coconut flour
- 1 tablespoon granulated sweetener
- 1/4 tsp salt
- 5 tablespoons butter cooled and cut into small pieces
- 2-4 tbsp fill with water
- 1/2 cup almond come Class
- 6 tablespoons chocolate
- 1 teaspoon sweetener

- 2 large eggs
- 5 tablespoons water
- 1/4 cup melted butter
- 1 tablespoon Sorkin fiber syrup (optional, but helps create a gooier center)
- 1/2 teaspoon vanilla
- 3 tablespoons sugar-Free Chocolate Chips

Topping:

- 1 cup Light Whipping Cream
- 2 Tbsp Confectioners Sweetener
- 1/4 teaspoon Vanilla
- 1/2 Ounce Sugar -Free Bitter
- Chocolate

Instructions

Crust:

- Oven The 3 Preheat at 25F and grease a glass or ceramic pie pan.
- In a large bowl, mix almond flour, coconut flour, sweetener, and salt. Cut a pastry cutter or two sharp knives into the butter until the mixture resembles coarse pieces. Add two tablespoons of water and blend until the dough comes out. Add more water until it becomes necessary to urge the dough to return together.

- Press evenly into the rock bottom and prick down the sides of the prepared pie pan, with the included edges and fork. Bake for 12 minutes.
- Filling: In a large bowl whisks together almond flour, chocolate, sweetener, and leaven. Stir in eggs, water, melted butter, and vanilla until well combined. Stir in the chocolate chips.
- Pour batter into the crust and bake for half an hour, covering with foil halfway through. Remove and let cool for 10 minutes, then refrigerate for half an hour until cooled.

Topping:

- Mix cream, sweetener, and vanilla during a large bowl. Beat until cream holds stiff peaks. Cover cold filling.
- Shave the chocolate on top. Chill for an hour or two until completely set.

Easy Lemon With Coconut Milk

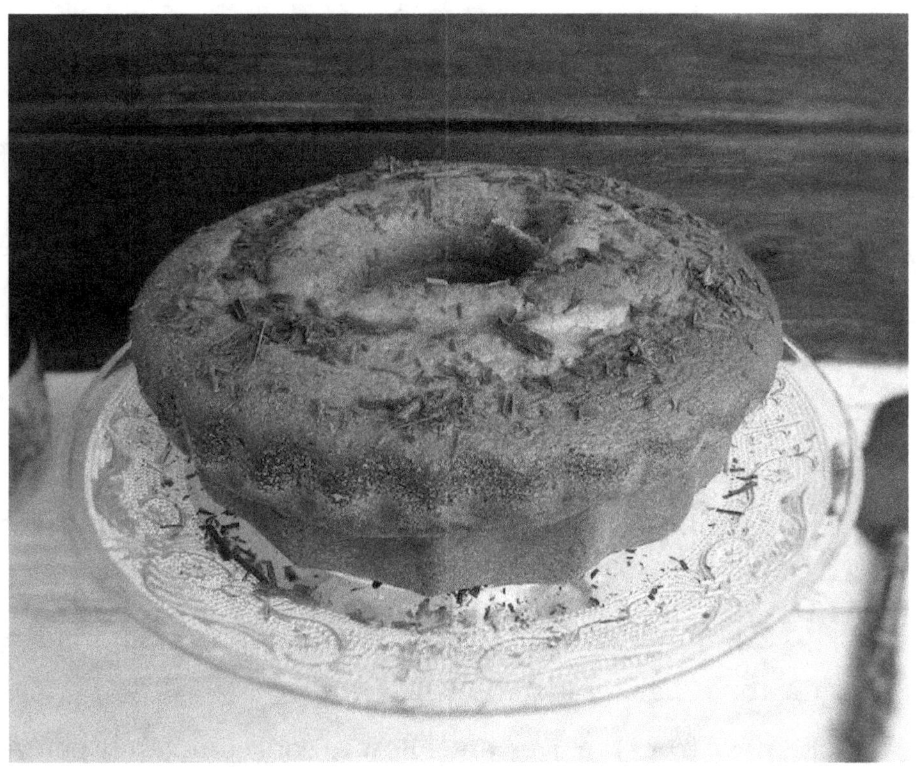

Ingredients

- 2 large eggs can use 3 for stiffer custard
- 1 cup coconut milk canned
- low cup low carb sugar substitute 1/2 cup preferred
- a cup coconut flour
- 2 tablespoons butter melted and free of oil dairy for cooling (use butter flavored copra)
- 1 teaspoon vanilla
- ¾ teaspoon yeast

- 1 teaspoon lemon peel
- ½ teaspoon flavor
- 4 oz image available Shredded Coconut

Instructions

- Spray a 9-inch pie dish with cooking spray and preheat the oven to 350 degrees.
- In a large bowl, combine eggs, coconut milk, sweetener, coconut flour, butter, yeast, vanilla, lemon rind, and flavor. Stir until combined.
- Fold within the disgruntled coconut. Pour mixture into the pie dish.
- 40 - 45 minutes or until the arms turn brown and hence the top is light golden brown.
- Remove from the oven and allow to cool completely before cutting and serving.
- Store leftovers within the refrigerator for 3 days.

Sugar-Free Lemon Pie
(Low Carb and Grain Free)

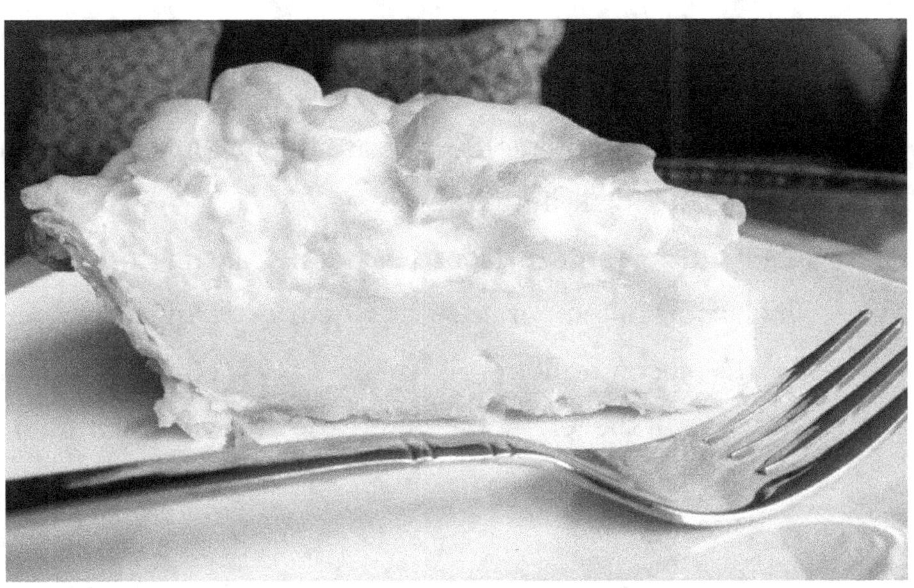

Ingredients

- Free Lemon Cheese
- 1/2 cup juice or about 5 small lemon juice ingredients - Put the Marin
- 2 eggs
- 1/2 cup butter or copra oil,
- melt 1/4 cup erythritol -erythritol or monk fructose
- soft sugar-free meringue frosting tag
- 2 egg white
- 1/4 cup erythritol

Instructions

- Whisk juice, sweetener, eggs and egg yolk together during a saucepan.

- Bring to medium heat and add oil or butter, stirring constantly, to cook and avoid scrambling eggs.

- When the copra oil melts, increase the heat from medium to high, stirring it until it thickens.

- When thick, remove from heat and transfer to a bowl, which cools to temperature for a quarter of an hour.

- Fill the coconut flour pie inside the shell with lemon flower. Chill the lemon pie to settle for at least 2 hours.

Before Serving:

- In a bowl, whisk the album until it starts producing an honest volume, usually 30 seconds at high speed.

- Keep whispering at a fast pace and slowly add the sugar-free crystal sweetener of your choice.

- After 1 minute and 30 seconds, the meringue should be fluffy and triple its volume.

- Above the bowl to see if the meringue is ready. If it sticks with bowl transfer to the highest of the lemon cheese pie.

- Place the top of the flame on the torch or grill inside the oven for 2 minutes until the highest is slightly brown.

- Sugar-Free Crystal Sweetener: You will use Saver in Native or Monk Fructose or Erythritol in the US / Canada, New Zealand, and Australia.

- Meringue Replacement: If you don't have time to make the meringue, serve the pie with a sprinkling of uncooked coconut or fresh strawberries on top!

Pan: I have used an 8-inch loose bottom pan for this recipe.

Chayote Squash Mock Pie

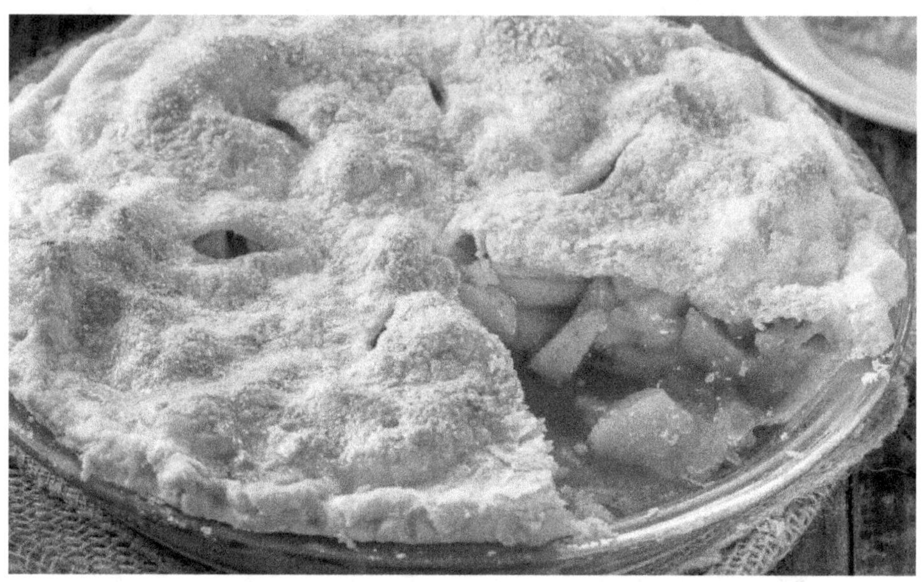

Ingredients

Crust:

- 1/2 cup butter melted
- 1 1/2 cups almond flour
- 3/4 cup coconut flour
- 4 eggs
- 1 tbsp whole onion
- 1/2 teaspoon salt

Filling:

- 5 medium chayote squash
- 3/4 cup Substitute low carb sugar

- 1 1/2 teaspoon cinnamon
- 1/4 teaspoon ginger
- 1/8 teaspoon nutmeg
- 1 tbsp xanthan gum
- 1 tbsp juice
- 2 tablespoons apple extract optional
- 1/3 cup butter cut. Small pieces

Topping:

- 1 egg
- low carb sugar substitute

Instructions

Crust:

- Mix crust ingredients to make the dough.
- Separate into two dough balls.
- Roll each crust ball into a pie shell.
- Transfer a crust to a 9-inch pie dish. Smooth out any cracks.
- The remaining crust reserved for the pie top.

Fill:

- Peel chayote and slice digging.
- Boil chopped chayote until fork tender. drain. Return to the vessel.

- Add cinnamon, ginger, nutmeg, sweetener, xanthan gum, juice, and apple extracts to the cooked chia squash.
- Pour the chayote mixture into the prepared pie shell. Fill with butter.

Topping:

- Cover filling with the preserved pie shell.
- Mix the sides of the pie shell and cut the slits on the pie top.
- If desired, brush the top crust and sprinkle with additional sweetener.
- Bake at 375 ° F for 30-35 minutes (I took me out after 30 minutes).

Chapter 8: Shakes & Smoothies Recipes

Sugar-Free Flavored Frappuccino

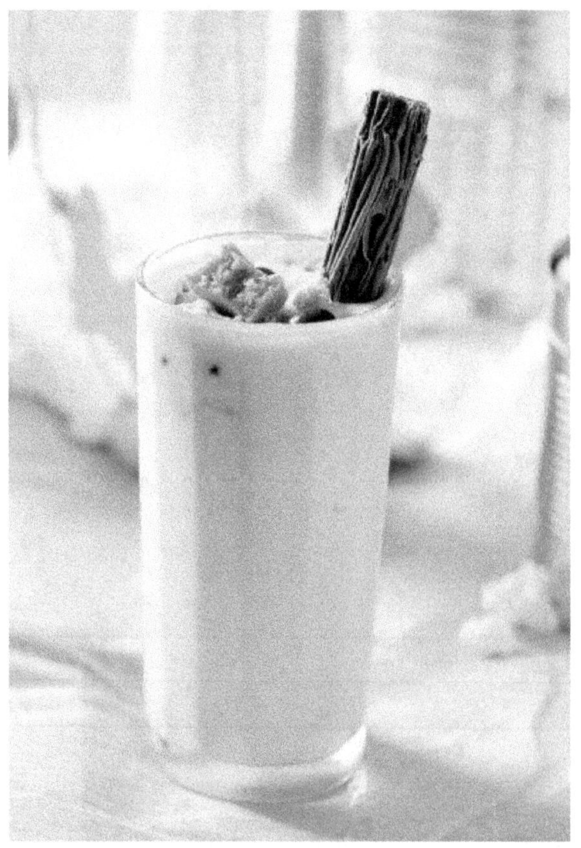

Ingredients

- 2 cups Vanilla Almond Milk
- 1 cup Heavy Light Cream

- Whipping 1 Flavor or 1 tsp Vanilla Split wise Unsaturated and
- 1/2 1/2 teaspoon Vanilla Liquid Stevia
- 2 cups Ice
- Optional Topping: Topping Chocolate Shaving
- 1/4. tsp xanthan for alternating glue

Instructions

- Keep all the ingredients together except ice.
- Blend on high for just a few seconds to blend.
- Add ice and mix again for just a moment to crush the ice.
- Taste and adjust the stevia if necessary.
- Serves about 1 1/2 cups each of 4 or serves 2 for a larger portion!

Keto Cookies and Cream Milkshake

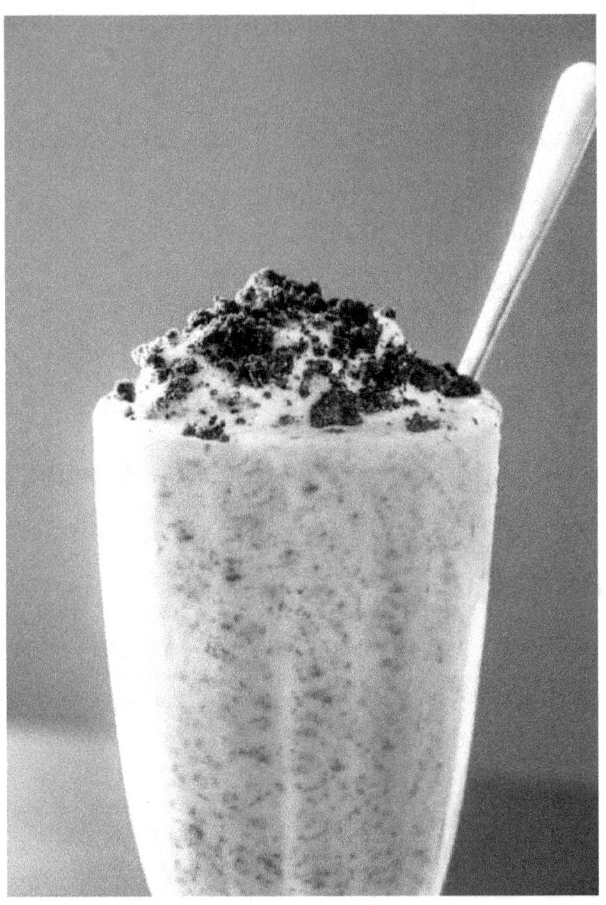

Ingredients

(2 servings)

- 3/4 cup Heavy Light Whipping Cream or Coconut Milk (180 ml / 6 oz)

- 1 cup uncooked almond milk or any nuts or seeds Milk (240 ml / 8 FL oz)

- 2 tablespoons almond butter, preferably roasted or edible seed butter (32 g / 1.1 oz)
- 1 tsp vanilla powder or sugar-free vanilla
- 1-2 tsp erythritol powder
- 3 cups chopped Walnuts or Pecans (40) g / 1.4 Us)
- glowing chocolate (at least 85%), grated (20 g / 2 largeo.7
- a few pieces of ice or almond Duke Frozen cubes
- forgoing 2 Spoon Topping or Coconut Milk

Instructions

- Place all ingredients except for the smoothie (which you serve for topping) until a high-speed blender and blitz smooth together. The blitz the longer you thicken it. Just be happy to beat the blitz once or reserve some grated chocolate, walnuts and almond butter for the topping.
- In another bowl, which elevates the cream for topping. For a straight beat, use at least half to 1 cup of cream. Any remaining toppings are often kept within the fridge during a sealed jar for up to three days.
- Pour into the shaking glass and top each with a large spoon of topping. Sprinkle with reserved grated chocolate, crumbled walnuts, and drizzle with leftover almond butter. Taste best when served fresh.

Low Carb Almond Butter Smoothie

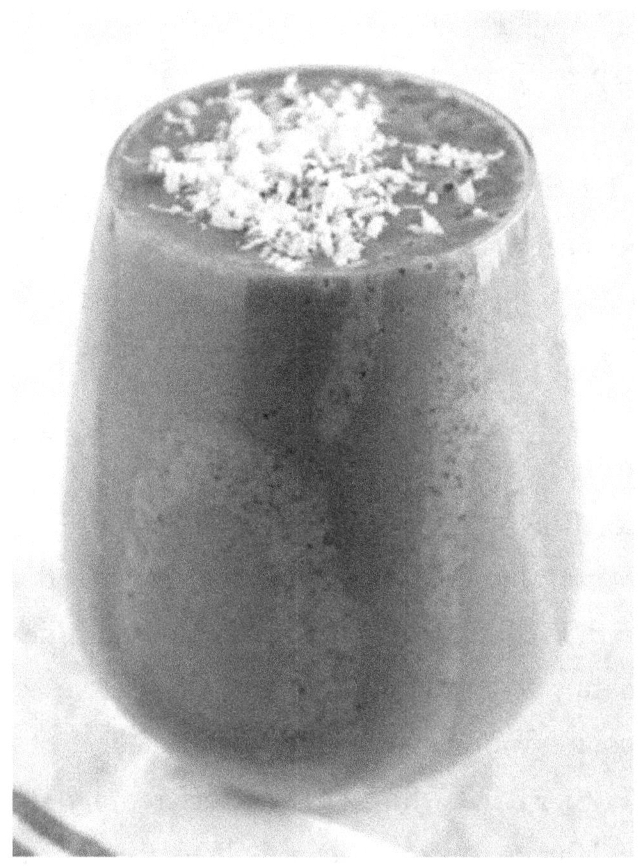

Ingredients

- 1 100g Pack Unsaturated Acai Puree
- 3/4 cup Unsweetened Almond Milk
- 1/4 of an Avocado
- 3 tala Collagen or Protein Powder
- 1 tbsp copra oil or MCT Oil Powder
- 1 tbsp almond butter

- 1/2 tsp vanilla.
- 2 drops liquid stevia (optional)

Instructions

- If you are using individual 100-gram packs of acai puree, stir the pack under lukewarm water for a few seconds until you can hack the puree into small pieces. Don't be ready to open the pack and pour the contents into the blender.
- Place the remaining ingredients within the blender and blend until smooth. Add more water or ice cubes as needed.
- Drizzle with almond butter along the edge of the glass to cool it down.
- Enjoy and pat yourself on the back for an awesome workout and killer post-workout thug!

Paleo & Keto Chocolate

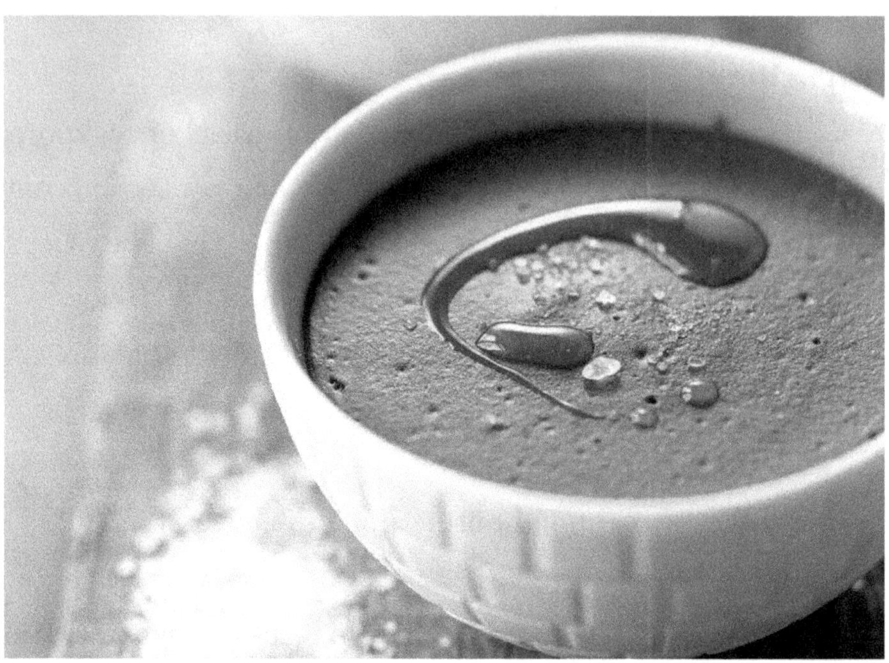

Ingredients

- 1/2 cup full-fat coconut milk or cream
- 1/2 medium avocado
- 1-2 tablespoons cocoa powder to taste
- 1/2 teaspoon vanilla
- pinch pink Himalayan salt and salt of choice
- 2-4 tablespoons erythritol or the sweetener like, to taste
- as Ashoke 1/2 cup ice
- Pinkie as required
- Optional add-ins

- Chia seeds ground (you've got to add more water
- MCT oil
- Hemp hearts
- Peptides collagen

Instructions.

- Put Coconut milk Jaehnig, avocado, cocoa powder, vanilla, salt, sweetener and add-ins option in a blender (tablets wonderful works are!) Here. Blend until the cream is smooth, employing a little water as needed.
- Add to ice and blend until thick and creamy. Do not over-mix, or you will lose thickness and coolness. Enjoy immediately!

Sugar-Free Keto Vanilla Milkshake

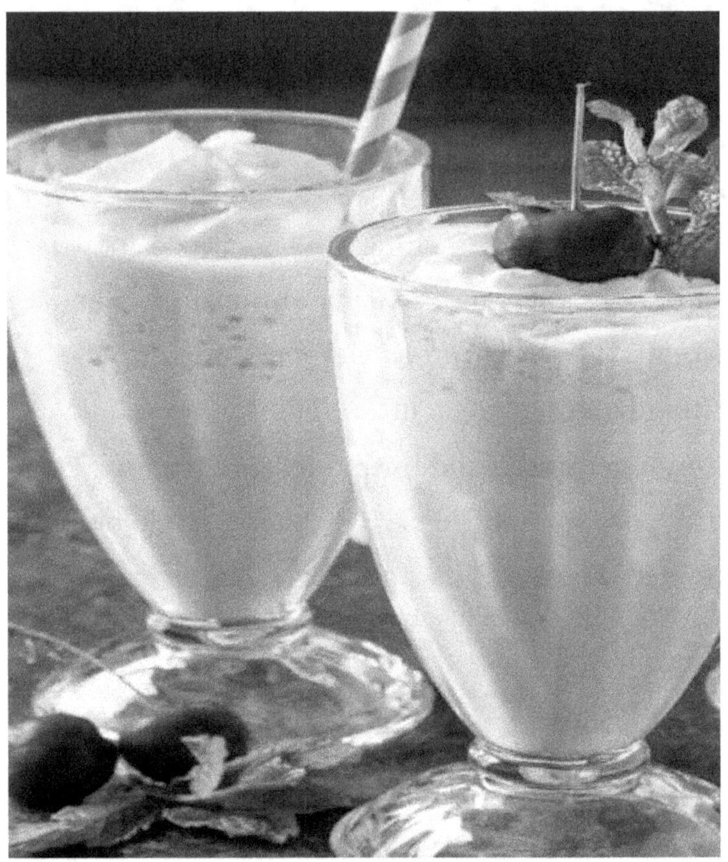

Ingredients

"Fancy" Version:

- wet cup uncooked almond milk (150ml))
- cup cream (100ml)
- ill vanilla pod
- sugar spoon sugar-free vanilla (leave to use silica-flavored sweetener to taste)

- liquid sweetener

- 5 ice cubes

Fast Version:

- us unsaturated cup almond milk (150ml) (150ml)

- cream cup cream (100ml)

- 1 teaspoon vanilla

- sugar-free flavor: liquid sweetener (a sugar-free vanilla syrup working here Singing!)

- Ice cubes

Instructions.

- Cut the vanilla pod in half and take out the seeds.

- Pour Cream into a little non-sticking pot and add vanilla seeds as well, because the pods are cream.

- Boil the cream while stirring continuously. (I like to recommend setting the heat to low-medium instead of high - this may reduce your chances of burning the cream).

- Remove the vanilla pod that has been sprinkled with cream and fill the infused cream in a jar or mug.

- Refrigerate in your fridge until cold (About 1 hour).

- Add vanilla-infused creams and each of the remaining ingredients to the kitchen appliance and mix approx. 30 seconds.

- Confirm not to mix for too long because friction can heat your milkshake and I think we would all agree that a hot milkshake doesn't sound like something we want!

Fast version:

- Add all ingredients to a kitchen appliance and mix approx. 30 seconds.
- Confirm not to mix for too long because friction can heat your milkshake and I think we would all agree that a hot milkshake doesn't sound like something we want!

Conclusion

Thank you for making it through to the end of *Keto Desserts Cookbook*, let's hope it was informative and able to provide you with all of the tools you need to achieve your goals whatever they may be.

The Ketogenic diet is an effective and comparatively safe treatment of effective seizures. Despite its long history, however, much is known about the diet, including its methodology, optimal protocol, and, therefore, its full range of applicability. Dietary investigations are providing new insights into the mechanisms behind seizures and epilepsy, as well as possible new treatments.

Finally, if you found this book useful in any way, a review on Amazon is always appreciated!